Aspects of Midwifery Practice
A research-based approach

Edited by

Jo Alexander, Valerie Levy
and Sarah Roch

MACMILLAN

This volume is dedicated to the memory of
JANETTE BRIERLEY
a midwife who made an outstanding contribution to her
profession.
Janette died in 1993 and is greatly missed by her family,
friends and colleagues

Contents

Other volumes in the Midwifery Practice Series

Contributors to this volume

Elaine Carty RN, MSN, CNM
Associate Professor, School of Nursing, University of British Columbia and Associate Midwife, British Columbia Women's Hospital, Vancouver
Elaine Carty has published a number of articles on issues relating to disability and parenting. She is a co-ordinator for the University of British Columbia's Childbearing and Parenting Program for women with disabilities/chronic illnesses.

Terri Coates RN, RM, ADM, DipED
Distance Learning Tutor, South Bank University and Practising Midwife in Salisbury and Southampton
Until April 1994, Terri Coates was a Midwifery Tutor at The Princess Anne Hospital, Southampton. She wrote her ADM Dissertation on shoulder dystocia and has been lecturing extensively on the subject ever since.

Jo Garcia BA, MSc
Social Scientist, The National Perinatal Epidemiology Unit, Oxford
Jo Garcia is currently Acting Director of the Midwifery Research Programme at the NPEU. She has written widely and, in 1989, was co-editor of *The Politics of Maternity Care.*

Alan Jackson, MD, FRCP
Institute of Human Nutrition, University of Southampton
Alan Jackson is Professor of Human Nutrition, in the School of Biological Sciences at the University of Southampton.

Sally Marchant RN, RM, ADM, Diploma in Research Methods
Research Midwife, The National Perinatal Epidemiology Unit, Oxford
Sally Marchant is currently pursuing a programme of research into women's health postnatally, and focusing in particular upon bleeding in the postnatal period.

Carolyn Roth BA, SRN, SCM, PGCEA
Senior Lecturer in Midwifery Studies, South Bank University
Until March 1990, Carolyn Roth was a Midwifery Tutor at St Mary's Hospital London. Her responsibilities at Southbank University include that of Course Director for the BSc (Hons) in Midwifery Studies, the Diploma in Professional Studies in Midwifery and the MSc in Midwifery Studies.

Catherine Siney SRN, RM
Specialist Midwife (Drug Liaison), Liverpool Women's Hospital
Catherine Siney was involved in the setting up of provision of antenatal care and advice for female drug users in Liverpool in 1990. In 1992 she received the Nursing Standard Award (midwifery category) for this work. Her research interests include an investigation into the outcomes of pregnancy for opiate dependent women and the evaluation of a neonatal opiate withdrawal chart.

Jennifer Sleep BA, SRN, SCM, MTD
Director of Nursing and Midwifery Research, Berkshire College of Nursing and Midwifery
A contributor to Volumes 2 and 3 in this series, and to *Effective Care in Pregnancy and Childbirth,* Jennifer Sleep has been researching into and writing about perineal care for over a decade. She also co-ordinates nursing and midwifery research throughout the Berkshire Health Authority.

Susan L. Smith RGN, RM
Research Sister, Department of Neonatal Medicine, Princess Anne Hospital, Southampton and Co-ordinator for the Advanced Neonatal Nurse Practitioner Course (ENB A19)
The Research Sister element of Susan Smith's joint appointment enables her to be actively involved with babies, both in the neonatal unit and in the community. She is particularly interested in neonatal nutrition and in the further education of neonatal nurses.

Sally Spedding BSc(Hons), SRD
Chief Community Dietitian, Southampton University Hospitals NHS Trust
Sally Spedding has been working in Southampton for some years now and was appointed Chief Community Dietitian in April 1994.

Rosaline Steele BA, MA, RN, RM, ADM, MTD
Midwifery Education Co-ordinator, The Royal College of Midwives
An experienced midwifery teacher and practitioner, Rosaline Steele has a particular interest in supporting clinical midwives in the development of their practice.

Joan Wilson BSc(Hons), SRD
Senior 1 Paediatric Dietitian, Southampton University Hospitals NHS Trust
Joan Wilson's research interests include diet and pregnancy – the subject of her college thesis.

Sarah Wright BSc(Hons), SRD
Senior 1 Paediatric Dietitian, Southampton University Hospitals NHS Trust
Sarah Wright's previous clinical experience includes working with anaemic pregnant women in North Eastern Thailand.

Foreword

I am pleased to write this foreword for the next book in a popular series on midwifery practice with a research-based approach. Over the past five years midwives have owed much to the editors for bringing together such relevant and timely work regarding our everyday practice. This book – the fifth in the series is no exception.

In today's rapidly changing world it is, I believe, more important than ever before that midwives can speak up with confidence and authority on their work. They must be able to face any challenge with research-based knowledge. This book with its practice checks assists in linking the research evidence with everyday work.

All over the UK midwives are striving to deliver woman-centred care and this often means change. Midwives need to be equipped to take a lead in local and national debates on the future of the maternity services. This book will play a part in assisting those midwives and I welcome its publication.

Margaret Brain
DBE RN RM MTD FRCOG

Preface

With the publication and implementation of the 'Changing Childbirth' report (Expert Maternity Group 1993), many midwives are extending and developing their role and asserting their right to use the full range of their midwifery skills. In order to practise innovatively and safely, midwives need to be active and critical consumers of research. The purpose of this series of books is to provide quick and convenient access to research findings relating to clinical practice. Although the series is written primarily for midwives, we hope it may prove useful to other health care professionals and to consumers of the maternity services.

Within the midwifery profession over the past few years there has been an upsurge of interest and expertise in research. Midwives are participating in research methods courses, increasingly available by attendance or distance learning mode, in which the skills of accessing, evaluating and implementing research findings are developed. The increasing numbers of midwives undertaking research is evidenced by the expanding size of the MIRIAD (the Midwifery Research Database) publication, which continues to provide an essential reference to what studies are being, or have been, carried out, by whom and where. The Cochrane Collaboration Pregnancy and Childbirth Database supplies accessible and essential information on the randomised controlled trials concerning midwifery practice and is now readily available to any midwife who has access to a computer.

Despite these initiatives, research information is still not always easily accessible to midwives, and this series is intended to fill the vacuum. The series offers midwives and student midwives a broad ranging survey and analysis of the research literature relating to central areas of clinical practice. The books do not intend to provide the comprehensive coverage of a definitive textbook; indeed their strength derives from the in-depth treatment of a selection of topics. The topic areas were chosen with care and contributors (most, but not all, of whom are midwives) were approached who have a particular research interest and expertise. On the basis of their critical appraisal of the literature, the authors make recommendations for clinical practice, and thus the predominant feature of these books is the link made between research and key areas of practice.

The chapters have a common structure, identical to that found in previous volumes, and this is described below. Some knowledge of research terminology will prove useful but its lack should not discourage readers. Midwifery practice is always evolving as new research data become available, and this is certainly the case since the first volumes in the series were published in 1990. This volume contains two updated chapters from earlier volumes concerning key areas of practice – 'Postnatal perineal care revisited' and 'HIV in pregnancy', contributed by Jennifer Sleep and Carolyn Roth respectively.

We would like to express our gratitude to authors who have worked painstakingly to produce their contributions, to our publishers, and to Richenda Milton-Thompson who continues her invaluable role as publisher's editor for the series. Her skill and enthusiasm have contributed enormously to its success.

JA
VL
SR
November 1994

■ Common structure of the chapters

In fulfilment of the aims of the series, each chapter follows a common structure:

1. The introduction offers a digest of the contents;
2. *'It is assumed that you are already aware of the following ...'* establishes the prerequisite knowledge and experience assumed of the reader;
3. The main body of the chapter then reviews and analyses the most appropriate and important research literature currently available;
4. The *'Recommendations for clinical practice'* offer suggestions for sound clinical practice, based on the author's interpretation of the literature;
5. The *'Practice check'* enables professionals to examine their

own practice and the principles and policies influencing their work;
6. Bibliographic sources are covered under *References* and *Suggested further reading.*

■ Reference

Expert Maternity Group 1993 Changing childbirth. HMSO, London

■ Further reading on research

Burnard P, Morrison P 1994 Nursing research in action – developing basic skills, 2nd edn. Macmillan, Basingstoke
Cormack DFS (ed) 1991 The research process in nursing, 2nd edn. Blackwell Scientific Publications, Oxford
Distance Learning Centre packages 1988–1994 Research awareness: a programme for nurses, midwives and health visitors, Units 1–11. Southbank University, London
Field PA, Morse JM 1985 Nursing research: the application of qualitative approaches. Croom Helm, London
Hicks C 1990 Research and statistics: a practical introduction for nurses. Prentice Hall, Hemel Hempstead

Chapter 1

Nutrition for pregnancy and lactation

Sally Spedding, Joan Wilson, Sarah Wright, Alan Jackson

The biological objective of pregnancy is to produce a healthy baby, whilst at the same time assuring that the mother's health is protected, not least so that she can provide good quality breast milk to ensure the health of the baby for the first six months of life. This objective is most readily achieved by a woman who enjoys good health at the time when she becomes pregnant, is able to take a varied healthy diet, has a reasonable balance of rest and activity during the pregnancy, is able to avoid infections, and is a good size. Women of normal size (Body Mass Index between 20 and 25 kg per m^2) should, on average, gain 10–12.5 kg during pregnancy (HEA 1994). Women who are underweight need to gain more. Women who are overweight present a particular difficulty; it is important that they do not gain excessive weight. For most, maintaining their weight is to be preferred and for a woman who is very heavy there may be benefit of some weight loss during pregnancy, provided that at the same time an adequate intake of nutrients can be assured. It is obvious that the growing baby needs energy and nutrients to be able to grow properly and these have to be provided by a combination of the reserves already present in the mother at the time of conception and her intake over the course of the pregnancy. Any stress which competes for the energy and nutrients presents a risk to the baby. Thus the body of a young woman, still in the late stages of adolescence, or a woman who is underweight when pregnancy starts, requires more nutrients for her own body, setting up a competitive demand with the needs of the growing baby.

Although all nutrients are important in terms of meeting dietary

1

needs, those which have received particular attention in recent years are vitamin A, C, and D, folate, iron, calcium, protein, dietary fibre, and energy. Consequently, the literature which has been reviewed for this chapter focuses on these nutrients. Infection during pregnancy presents a risk of damage to the fetus, both directly and indirectly. In this context, food safety is of critical importance and is an issue about which the essential information can often be appropriately addressed in combination with dietary advice.

The following chapter discusses the research results which are available at the present time and the current recommendations for the nutrition of women during pregnancy and lactation in the United Kingdom. Particular emphasis has been placed upon issues of food safety and the nutrients identified above. Suggestions given for energy and nutrient intakes are referred to as 'reference values'. This is because they are estimates of 'Dietary Reference Values' (DoH 1991) and *not* recommendations for intakes by individuals or groups. Discussion of the Dietary Reference Values, and the role of nutrients not identified above, is beyond the scope of the present chapter, however an exploration of them is recommended as further reading.

The chapter aims to assist midwives in deciding what information to offer women about nutrition. People eat food as a source of enjoyment and pleasure, not simply as a source of nutrients. Therefore, a section is included which provides suggestions on the recommendations translated in terms of practical dietary advice.

■ **It is assumed that you are already aware of the following:**

- The basic physiology of pregnancy and lactation;
- The functions of different nutrients;
- Foods in which energy and nutrients are found;
- The main principles of 'healthy eating' in terms of high fibre, low fat, low sugar and low salt, and how to implement them in terms of food selection.

All DRVs are intended to apply to healthy people; they do not make any allowance for the different energy and nutrient needs imposed by some diseases.

Dietary Reference Values:
A general term used to cover all the figures produced by the Panel – LRNI, EAR, RNI and safe intake

Estimated Average Requirement (EAR):
The Panel's estimate of the average requirement or need for food energy or a nutrient. Clearly, many people will need *more* than the average and many people will need *less*

Reference Nutrient Intake (RNI):
An amount of a nutrient that is enough for almost every individual, even someone who has high needs for the nutrient. This level of intake, therefore, is considerably higher than most people *need*. If individuals are consuming the RNI of a nutrient, they are most unlikely to be deficient in that nutrient

Lower Reference Nutrient Intake (LRNI):
The amount of a nutrient that is enough for only the small number of people with *low* needs. Most people will need more than the LRNI if they are to eat enough. If individuals are habitually eating *less* than the LRNI they will almost certainly be deficient

Safe Intake:
A term normally used to indicate the intake of a nutrient for which there is not enough information to estimate requirements. A safe intake is one which is judged to be adequate for almost everyone's need but not so large as to cause undesirable effects

By using the term 'reference', the Panel hoped that users will not interpret any of the figures as *recommended* or desirable intakes but will use the most appropriate set of figures for any given situation and use them as a general point of reference rather than as definitive values set in tablets of stone.

Taken from Dietary Reference Values: A guide (DoH 1991)

Figure 1.1 Dietary reference values (DRVs)

■ Nutritional needs during pregnancy and lactation

□ Energy

Pregnancy The extent to which there is the need for a substantial increase in energy intake during pregnancy for women in the UK has recently been critically reassessed. The theoretical energy costs are due to growth and other changes in maternal and fetal tissues, and an increase in Basal Metabolic Rate (BMR), which together come to a total of about 250–300 kcalories per day (Hytten & Leitch 1971). There is little doubt that pregnancy represents an increased demand of this order, but the need might be satisfied in a number of different ways: from body reserves, an increase in dietary intake, or a decrease in physical activity, or any combination of the three. Recent evidence has suggested that, at the present time, the level of physical activity of pregnant women decreases which leads to a saving in energy. The result is that the energy saved can be used to support the pregnancy and therefore there is less need for the dietary intake to increase (Durnin 1991). Based upon this information it has been concluded that a relatively small addition to the pre-pregnant energy intake should be adequate for the extra energy needs of the pregnant mother. Hence, the current recommendation is that a normal pregnant woman, living in an industrialised country, requires no more than an extra 100–150 kcal per day during the second and third trimester (DoH 1991). No extra kcalories are required during the first trimester.

There are two important consequences to this recommendation. Firstly, it is based upon the observation that women are relatively inactive, but there are undoubtedly health benefits to a balanced pattern of activity and rest during pregnancy. Were a woman to be more active she would require a greater intake of energy. Secondly, as energy intake is an important determinant of the total food intake, increasing intake as a result of increased activity is one important way in which the intake of all nutrients can be increased.

Lactation Chronic, severe undernutrition in the mother has been associated with poor lactational performance, represented by a reduced volume of breast milk, but milder forms of undernutrition appear to have a more modest effect, if any, on milk output (Whitehead 1983; Coward *et al* 1984). For example it has been shown in experimental studies, that when mothers, who are otherwise well nourished, were consuming 1500 kcal per day there was no significant reduction in milk output. With more severe caloric restriction, however, milk output was reduced, but the effect was delayed (Butte *et al* 1984). On 1500 kcal per day, the mothers lost weight and it appeared as though milk volume was protected at the expense of maternal reserves. It was estimated that an energy intake of approximately 2600 kcal per day would be required to support lactation whilst maintaining maternal weight. Strode and colleagues (1986) have suggested that an intake of 2215 kcal per day results in weight loss in well nourished mothers whilst supporting an acceptable rate of infant growth, similar to reference standards. During pregnancy maternal weight is gained and it is assumed that this is a protection against the increased demands of lactation. Therefore, some weight loss during lactation is seen as desirable. It has been shown that a weight loss of 0.5 kg per week by mothers during lactation has no obvious adverse effects on the mother or the infant (Strode *et al* 1986). Current estimated average requirements (EAR) for energy intake during lactation has been set at 2180–2510 kcal per day for mothers aged 19–50 years (DoH 1991).

□ **Protein**

Pregnancy Protein is required for the elaboration of maternal and fetal tissues. Although the increased intake over the entire pregnancy is substantial (900 g), on a daily basis this is only about 3 g per day (Hytten & Leitch 1971). The habitual protein intake of non-pregnant women in the UK is about 62 g per day on average, with about 12 per cent of women taking less than 45 g per day (Gregory *et al* 1990). The current reference intake of protein for pregnant women is an additional 6 g protein per day on the reference nutrient intake (RNI) of a non-pregnant woman (45 g per day) to a total of 51 g per day for pregnant women aged 19–50 years (DoH 1991). Therefore it would appear that, for the majority of women, as the habitual intake of protein is generous, the additional demands of pregnancy can be met with no further increase. There may, however, be a group of women who require special attention on an individual basis.

There is no evidence that high protein intakes, for example through the use of high protein supplements, confer any benefit. Indeed there is some concern that intakes of protein in excess of those normally taken in the UK may lead to damage by increasing the risk of low birthweight, preterm births and fetal renal damage (Schiffman *et al* 1989; Abrams & Berman 1993).

Lactation The protein which passes into breast milk places an obvious demand upon the maternal system. Milk protein output, however, varies with each stage of lactation (Butte *et al* 1984), maternal diet (Forsum & Lonnerdahl 1980) and nutritional status (Sanchez-Poso *et al* 1987). The international expert consultation (FAO/WHO/UNU 1985) proposed that the daily protein intake be increased by 0.3 g protein per kg maternal body weight, to 1.1 g protein per kg per day during lactation. This was based on the assumption that maternal protein requirements would be increased in proportion to the quantity of milk secreted during lactation. Experimental studies since that time have indicated that this might be an underestimate of the requirements. Thomas and colleagues (1991) concluded that a maternal intake of 1.3 g protein per kg per day was insufficient to support the protein needs of lactation. Another study from the same group (Children's Nutrition Research Centre 1991) found that, amongst a group of mothers who successfully breast fed their infants, the intake of protein naturally selected was 1.5 g protein per kg per day. There are no studies which provide evidence of a detrimental effect of a larger protein intake during lactation. At the present time the RNI in the UK to cover the requirements for lactation are 53–56 g protein for women aged 19–50 years (DoH 1991).

□ **Vitamin A**

Pregnancy Extra vitamin A is required for the growth and maintenance of the fetus, for fetal stores, and for maternal tissue growth (DoH 1991). At all ages (intra- and extrauterine life) there is normally a store of vitamin A in the liver. The ability of the unborn baby to develop its own store of vitamin A is profoundly affected by the nutritional status of the mother. If the vitamin A status of the mother herself is impaired, the development of fetal stores is compromised (Ganguly 1988). In the UK the risk is more likely to be from excessive intakes of vitamin A than from a deficiency. Excessive intakes of vitamin A in the periconceptual period or during early pregnancy have been shown to increase the risk of congenital abnormalities (DoH 1990). This is true whether the excess vitamin A is taken as an integral part of the diet or as a supplement. The risk is highest when the excessive intake is taken during the first two months of pregnancy (DoH 1990). Defects have been reported following the daily consumption of 25 000 international units, iu, (7500 μg per day) or more, over several weeks or months, whereas exposure to less than 10 000 iu per day are considered unlikely to be damaging to the fetus (Rosa *et al* 1986).

Multivitamin supplements which are specially designed for use in the prenatal period contain 5000 iu of vitamin A, or less. However, vitamin tablets which contain more than 25 000 iu can be obtained across the counter and may be taken by pregnant women. The Teratology Society (1975) recommend vitamin A supplementation during pregnancy should be limited to 8000 iu (2400 µg per day). The use of fish liver oil as a supplement is not recommended as it contains vitamin A in amounts which could provide a higher intake of vitamin A than found in multivitamin tablets (DoH 1990).

Recent concern has been expressed about the vitamin A content of some animal liver which may be available for general consumption. The vitamin A content of liver commonly available in the UK may range from 13 000 µg to 40 000 µg per 100 g (DoH 1991). The consumption of generous portions of liver containing the higher concentrations of vitamin A might expose women to potentially damaging levels of the vitamin. This raises the question of whether liver should be excluded from the diet of pregnant women. On the one hand there is the potential risk of damage from vitamin A toxicity. On the other, as pointed out by Doyle and colleagues (1989), there are limited ways in which low income families can achieve a nutritious diet. Many nutrients, deficiency of which have been implicated in increasing the risk of low birthweight – for example thiamin, riboflavin, niacin, zinc and iron, are all provided in relatively generous amounts at a low cost by liver. Nelson (1990) has argued that no more than 50 g liver per week or 100 g liver products (e.g. pâté) should be consumed until the vitamin A content of products is reduced. It could, therefore, be argued that liver need not be entirely excluded from the diet. The Department of Health (1990, 1993) has advised that, as a precautionary measure, women who are pregnant, or might become pregnant, should not take excessive quantities of vitamin A, and should not consume liver or liver products. The RNI for vitamin A is a modest increase of 100 µg of vitamin A daily above the non-pregnant requirement of 600 µg per day (for a woman aged 19–50 years) (DoH 1991). In the USA, the National Research Council (the advisory body on dietary allowances) has recommended that if a supplement is required for recent immigrants from countries where vitamin A deficiency is endemic or for those with a demonstrably inadequate diet, then it should be given in the form of β-carotene (4800 µg) which can be converted to vitamin A in the body, as this is unlikely to produce vitamin A toxicity (Obstetrics Committee 1993).

Lactation   The milk produced by well nourished mothers contains a relatively large amount of vitamin A. The current recommendations, therefore, suggest that during lactation an increased intake of 350 µg per day, should bring the total vitamin A reference intake to 950 µg per day for a woman aged 19–50 years (DoH 1991).

☐ **Folic acid (folate)**

Pregnancy Since 1964, there has been evidence to suggest that a less than optimal level of folic acid in a woman in the periconceptual period is one important factor which might increase the risk of the development of neural tube defect (NTD) in a developing fetus (Hibbard & Smithells 1965). Conclusive evidence for the effect has been difficult to come by, although a number of studies were set up with this as their objective. For example, women who have already had one child with NTD are at increased risk in subsequent pregnancies that the baby will have NTD, and this risk of recurrence could be reduced if a supplement of folic acid, with or without other vitamins, was taken around the time of conception. Laurence and colleagues (1981) gave women at increased risk a 4 mg daily supplement of folic acid, but the study had too few participants to provide a definitive answer. Smithells *et al* (1983) used a multivitamin preparation containing a mixture of eight vitamins including 0.36 mg of folic acid as a supplement, however because of the study's design the possibility that bias had been introduced could not be excluded. In 1985 a carefully designed, international, collaborative trial was set up by the Medical Research Council. The numbers in the study were sufficient to provide clear results which showed that in women who had had a previous child with NTD a supplement of 4 mg folic acid per day, starting preconceptionally, reduced the risk of a recurrence in a subsequent pregnancy by about 70 per cent. When the RNI for folic acid during pregnancy was set, 100 µg per day was added to the 200 µg per day for non-pregnant women aged 19 to 50 years, to give a total of 300 µg per day (DoH 1991). Since that time an Expert Advisory Group on Folic Acid (1992) has reviewed this advice in the light of the newer evidence relating to the association between folic acid and NTD. The recommendation from this group is that all women at risk of becoming pregnant should have an intake of folic acid of 400 µg per day, and that for those women at special risk, for example because they have a previously affected child, the recommendation is for 4 mg per day (4000 µg per day). This level of intake should be taken before conception and up to the twelfth week of pregnancy. It is possible to reach an intake of 400 µg per day by taking a diet rich in folate (for example by eating foods which are naturally rich in folate, such as green leafy vegetables like brussel sprouts, broccoli or spinach, or by taking foods which have been fortified with folate, such as breakfast cereals or enriched flour products). However, a special effort is required and therefore as a precautionary measure the Department of Health recommends that, at the present time, it would be prudent for all women who are planning a pregnancy to take a supplement of 400 µg folic acid. Those women at special risk, who require an intake of 4 mg per day, will need to take a high dose supplement, which is only available at the present time on prescription (in some areas the only available tablets may be of 5 mg dosage). The need for monitoring the effect of the recommendations was also emphasised (Expert Advisory Group 1992).

Lactation During lactation the reference nutrient intake includes an additional 60 µg per day, to compensate for incomplete absorption and utilisation of folate from the diet (DoH 1991).

□ **Vitamin C (ascorbic acid)**

Pregnancy Health food enthusiasts are especially keen to extol the virtues of vitamin C and there has been a tendency for very large supplements to be taken by certain groups. The evidence from an animal study has suggested a complex interaction between ascorbic acid and iron which strikes a note of caution. Although a high ascorbic acid intake during pregnancy has been found to enhance tissue ascorbate levels and iron stores in the mother, when combined with a high iron intake there was a reduction in the rate of growth of the offspring during the early stages of development in experimental animals (Bates *et al* 1988). Care has to be taken in extrapolation to humans, but certainly the evidence reinforces earlier views that caution should be exercised before any recommendation for the safety of supplementation with ascorbic acid can be made (Montgomery 1993).

The current reference nutrient intake assumes a moderate increase in requirement, especially in the final stages of pregnancy, as the fetus concentrates the vitamin at the expense of maternal stores and circulatory levels. This translates to an extra 10 mg per day, therefore a pregnant woman aged 19–50 years requires 50 mg vitamin C per day throughout pregnancy (DoH 1991).

Lactation There is little clear evidence about the influence of maternal intake of vitamin C on its subsequent concentration in human milk and infantile intake. Byerley and Kirksey (1985) studied 25 lactating women, who received various levels of supplementation with vitamin C. Subsequently the vitamin C content in breast milk and urine was assessed. The findings indicated an upper level to the concentration of vitamin C in milk, regardless of the level of supplementation, suggesting that a regulatory mechanism may be present in mammary cells to prevent an elevation beyond an upper limit. Dietary supplementation would only be expected to have an effect if the level of vitamin C in milk were below this critical level.

The current RNI for vitamin C is based upon an extra 30 mg per day (totalling 70 mg per day for a lactating woman aged 19–50 years). This should ensure the maintenance of adequate stores in the mother and levels in breast milk in the upper half of the normal range (DoH 1991). There is no evidence to date that intakes in excess of this confer any benefit (Montgomery 1993).

□ Vitamin D

Pregnancy The relationship between the maternal vitamin D and calcium status and that of the fetus is complex. It is well known that problems of bone growth in the mother, seen as short stature or frank rickets, may inhibit her ability to carry a successful pregnancy. However, it is less clear what can be done immediately before, or during pregnancy itself if the mother shows signs of such problems.

The only form of the vitamin D actively involved in calcium balance is 1,25-dihydroxy vitamin D (dihydroxy D), which is normally formed in the kidney, but may also be formed in the placenta during pregnancy. Dihydroxy D functions like a hormone and works by increasing both absorption of calcium from within the intestine and by releasing calcium from bone by resorption (Wilson *et al* 1990). In the normal course of events a substantial proportion of the body's requirement for vitamin D can be supplied by formation in the skin during exposure to sunlight (DoH 1991). It is not clear the extent to which the increased needs during pregnancy can be met through this route. Sunlight may be restricted in northern climates or for individuals in whom skin exposure is limited. After correcting for dietary intakes and level of exposure to sunlight, the serum levels of vitamin D during pregnancy do not seem to differ from that of the non-pregnant state and show the same seasonal variation

(Cockburn *et al* 1980; Beyers *et al* 1986). Serum levels of the active dihydroxy D have been found to be higher during pregnancy (Bouillon *et al* 1981; Wilson *et al* 1990). The stimulus for this increase is unknown. Delvin and colleagues (1986) have shown that, in women receiving supplementation with vitamin D, there appears to be a beneficial effect on perinatal handling of calcium, thereby preventing the possible occurrence of nutrition related rickets.

The RNI for vitamin D recommends that pregnant women should receive supplementary vitamin D to achieve an intake of 10 μg per day (DoH 1991).

Lactation Rickets caused by vitamin D deficiency in breast fed infants is now rarely reported in industrialised countries (Bhowmick *et al* 1991). Data regarding vitamin D status during lactation is still controversial. Greer and colleagues (1982) reported an increased maternal serum level of active vitamin D during lactation, however Wilson *et al* (1990) found a decrease in levels during the first two weeks of lactation. The available data suggest that as lactation proceeds an increased calcium demand may result in some elevation of the vitamin D levels. As in pregnancy, the advice for lactation remains that it is prudent to achieve a total intake of 10 μg per day (DoH 1991).

□ **Calcium**

Pregnancy The calcium needed for skeletal development of the fetus *in utero* means that there is inevitably a significant movement of calcium from the mother. There is little evidence to suggest that this is achieved by a spontaneous increase in the consumption of calcium by the pregnant woman. Rather, the evidence would favour the occurrence of an alteration of maternal calcium homeostasis (Purdie 1989). There are observations which indicate that there is an increase in the intestinal absorption of calcium during pregnancy (Heaney & Skillman 1971; Kent *et al* 1991). However, the hormonal mechanism which underlies the changes in calcium balance during the period of increased demand for calcium are still poorly understood (Misra & Anderson 1990). There is evidence that maternal bone density diminishes in the first trimester of pregnancy, suggesting that this reservoir is being drawn upon, but this appears to be replenished by six months postnatally (Purdie 1989).

The RNI for calcium during pregnancy has not been set at a level which is different to that in the non-pregnant state for healthy females aged 19–50 years, that is 700 mg per day. During adolescence, when there is still the need to satisfy the demand created by the growth of the mother's own bones, it would be desirable to have an extra 100 mg of calcium, making the RNI 800 mg daily (DoH 1991).

Lactation Circumstantial evidence suggests that there is adaptation in maternal calcium metabolism during lactation. To date, however, the information is not sufficient to make clear recommendations. Kent and colleagues (1991), showed that the absorption of calcium might be raised significantly in late pregnancy, but not during established lactation. As for most lactating women there is a spontaneous increase in food intake, it is desirable to ensure that this contributes to providing the additional 550 mg calcium per day which is needed for milk production. This brings the total reference intake of calcium during lactation to 1250 mg for a woman aged 19–50 years (DoH 1991).

□ **Iron**

Pregnancy Iron deficiency and iron deficiency anaemia are considered to be amongst the most common nutritional problems in both the developed and the developing world. Significant iron deficiency undoubtedly increases the risk of an adverse outcome in pregnancy. The control of the body content of iron is exerted through limiting the amount of iron absorbed from the diet. In the non-pregnant state only 10–20 per cent of dietary iron might be absorbed and this can increase during late pregnancy to 75–90 per cent. However, because iron supplementation trials in pregnancy have not always been successful, and because supplementation with iron can cause problems in susceptible individuals, some care is needed in deciding how best to approach the question of dietary and supplemental iron in pregnancy. The role of iron during pregnancy has been extensively reviewed by Montgomery (1993). The total increase in the requirement for iron to carry through a successful pregnancy has been estimated to be around 680 mg (Committee on Iron Deficiency 1968). In a woman who was previously adequately nourished this amount has the potential to be met from sources of iron already within the body, recognising that there is some saving in the losses of iron because of the cessation of menstruation, the ability to mobilise maternal stores, and the ability to increase intestinal absorption (Svanberg *et al* 1975; DoH 1991; Whittaker *et al* 1991). On this basis the routine supplementation of all women with iron has been considered unnecessary (DoH 1991; Montgomery 1993). However, there are women in whom the stores are too low at the start of pregnancy, and under these circumstances supplementation may be necessary. It is considered desirable to determine the iron status of the woman, which should include an assessment of iron stores (by the measurement of plasma ferritin), before supplementation is started (Montgomery 1993).

Lactation The current RNI for iron during lactation was based upon the finding of Vuori (1979) that iron concentrations in breast milk are 0.4 mg per litre between six and eight weeks postpartum, falling to 0.29 mg per litre between 17 and 22 weeks postpartum. It is generally assumed that 850 ml milk is produced daily, resulting in 0.25–0.34 mg per day of iron. This level of requirement may be offset by the saving in losses of iron associated with amenorrhoea, and therefore there is no reason to recommend an increase in intake (DoH 1991).

■ Nutritional considerations

□ Avoiding constipation

The hormonal changes which take place during pregnancy may affect the function of a wide range of tissues. Amongst these changes is a reduction in the motility of the gastrointestinal tract which leads to prolonged transit times (Hytten 1983). For this reason it is important to consider how changes in the diet might contribute to the prevention and/or treatment of constipation during pregnancy. The two changes which are most likely to confer benefit in the management of constipation are an increase in the consumption of 'dietary fibre' (or, more precisely, non-starch polysaccharides) and an increase in fluid intake (DoH 1991).

□ Food safety

Any infection in the mother will have a general effect on her body which might act to the disadvantage of the fetus. In addition, there are specific problems relating to microorganisms which are especially associated with food and therefore have relevance to dietary practice.

Listeriosis The illness listeriosis, which is caused by a common bacterium *Listeria monocytogenes* (Lm), is particularly dangerous during pregnancy. The condition attracted attention when it was identified as the cause of a series of cases of miscarriages, still-births and neonatal deaths (Caird 1989; DoH 1989; Quentin *et al* 1990). Prior to this increased publicity, it had been shown that Lm could be isolated from the faeces of 1 in 60 pregnant women and from 2 in 54 non-pregnant women (Lamont & Postlethwaite 1986). This indicated that pregnancy in itself was unlikely to increase the carriage rate of Lm. It is suggested that transmission of Lm probably occurs in one of four ways: trans-placental, as an ascending infection from the vagina, from the mother's genital tract during delivery, or after delivery due to cross infection (Carr & Rothburn 1989). Lm, a gram positive cocco bacillus, is widely distributed in the environment, e.g. soil, water and vegetation, therefore some exposure to it is unavoid-able (DoH 1989). Lm can multiply at temperatures which may be found in refrigerators (6°C or above). Fortunately, in most foods where it is present as a contaminant, it occurs at very low bacterial counts and is killed by adequate cooking times (DoH 1989). High counts of Lm have been found in some soft cheeses, fresh and frozen poultry, samples of pre-cooked, ready-to-eat poultry and cook-chill meals (Pini & Gilbert 1988; Gilbert *et al* 1989). Therefore, the current advice is that pregnant women should avoid soft, ripened cheeses, such as brie, camembert and blue vein types. They should also reheat ready-to-eat poultry and cook-chilled meals (purchased at retail outlets) until they are piping hot (DoH 1989; 1992).

Salmonella Although salmonellosis may have no direct effect on the fetus, the formal advice is that all (including pregnant women) should use extra care when handling and preparing poultry, raw meat and eggs to avoid contamination (DoH 1988; 1992). Eggs should be thoroughly cooked until the white and yolk are solid, and if following a recipe requiring partially cooked eggs, pas-teurised eggs should be used instead. Meat and poultry should be thoroughly cooked before eating. Raw meat should be kept separate from cooked meat to avoid cross-contamination.

Toxoplasmosis Toxoplasmosis, caused by the organism *Toxoplasma gondii*, has been found in raw meat and cat faeces, and can cause a mild flu-like illness in pregnant women and a range of prob-lems in the fetus (DoH 1992). Pregnant women are, therefore, advised to cook meat thoroughly and to remove soil and dirt from vegetables and salads. Goats' milk may also carry *Toxoplasma*, therefore pregnant women are advised not to consume untreated goats' milk (DoH 1992).

Milk-borne infections To reduce the risk of milk-borne infections, the Department of Health (1992) advise that pregnant women should avoid all milk which has not been heat-treated.

□ **Preconceptional considerations**

There is a relationship between birthweight and infant mortality. With falling birthweight, the prevalence of neurological and other handicaps increases dramatically (Winick *et al* 1975; OPCS 1988). Studies related to low birthweight (Kramer 1987; Doyle *et al* 1990; Wynn *et al* 1991) indicate that, in developed countries, prevention of low birthweight should focus on modifiable risk factors, such as smoking, diet and nutrition before and during pregnancy, very young maternal age, and maternal education. The results of research demonstrate that the availability of nutrients during the embryonic period can be critical for the wellbeing of healthy offspring (Giroud 1973).

Preconception care is about minimising risks. Women who have had a previous low birthweight infant face similar risks in subsequent pregnancies (Niswander & Gordon 1972) and, therefore, could be targeted for preconceptional nutrition advice whilst still receiving postnatal care. Low maternal pre-pregnant weight, which may reflect poor nutritional status, should also be addressed. One study in the UK has shown that, for a woman with a BMI below 19 kg per m², there is a threefold increase in the risk of having an infant who is small for dates (Van der Spuy *et al* 1988). As women who are underweight are at greater risk for a complicated pregnancy and more likely to produce a small baby, they are best advised to postpone conception until their BMI exceeds 19 kg per m². Active steps should be taken to advise how an increase in BMI might best be achieved by eating a healthy diet. It has been suggested that a BMI of around 24 kg per m² might be considered optimal for conception and pregnancy outcome (Wynn & Wynn 1990).

Close birth spacing may not allow some mothers time to recover from the nutritional demands of a previous pregnancy. This is because the placenta has the ability to concentrate, and thus considerably diminish, a number of vitamins including folate from the mother's circulation. The result is that the mother becomes depleted with low or marginal levels at the end of pregnancy. For example, it may take up to two years after pregnancy before iron depletion is restored and pre-pregnancy iron levels are regained (Worthington-Roberts *et al* 1989). Women taking oral contraceptive agents may have reduced plasma levels of vitamins, including thiamin, riboflavin, B_6, B_{12}, folate, and vitamin C, therefore some other form of contraception should be used in the preconceptional period to enable vitamin levels to normalise (British Dietetic Association 1993). Adolescent mothers are at increased risk of having preterm and low birthweight infants (Schonberg 1989), as the nutritional needs of pregnancy are in addition to those caused by the mother's physiological development. These mothers should, therefore, be targeted for nutritional advice. Excessive alcohol can affect the quality and quantity of sperm, as well as damaging the fetus, however no safe level of alcohol has yet been defined. For this reason it is advised that alcohol intake is minimised, if not avoided, when planning a pregnancy (Sulaiman *et al* 1988; Verkerk *et al* 1993).

Recent evidence suggests that nutrition may be an important environmental influence on the programming of the body's structure, physiology, and metabolism during fetal life, subsequently determining the risk in adult life of developing certain diseases, including cardiovascular disease and diabetes (Barker 1992; Barker *et al* 1993). The implications of this work, and the consequent practical recommendations for nutrition preconceptionally and during pregnancy, have yet to be defined, although it does indicate that achieving and maintaining optimal nutrition preconceptionally and during pregnancy may be more important than was initially thought.

■ Recommendations for clinical practice in the light of currently available evidence

1. On a regular basis, careful assessment should be made of mothers' dietary habits throughout all stages of pregnancy and lactation. At the time of writing practical tools are being developed to undertake this.
2. Every opportunity should be taken to promote a healthy diet, particularly for adolescent mothers.
3. Dietary recommendations should be based on current advice from the Department of Health to ensure consistency:
   - Assuming that nutritional recommendations are being achieved pre-conceptionally, the additional nutritional requirements for *pregnancy* can be met as follows:

- energy and protein – include an extra sandwich daily, consisting of bread and a protein filling;
- vitamin A and C – incorporate extra citrus fruit or fruit juice and extra vitamin A rich (generally orange/yellow coloured) fruit or vegetables into the diet;
- folate – supplement preconceptionally until the end of the first trimester, and encourage folate-rich foods, such as green, leafy vegetables and fortified breakfast cereals;
- Vitamin D – expose arms, face and legs to sunlight for 15–30 minutes daily, during summer months;
- 'Dietary fibre' – incorporate fruit, vegetables, and high fibre starchy foods. At least eight cups of fluid should be advised daily to prevent constipation.

• Assuming that nutritional recommendations have been achieved preconceptionally and during pregnancy, the extra nutritional needs of *lactation* (which are additional to those preconceptionally) can be met as follows:
- Calcium – include an extra pint of semi-skimmed milk into the diet daily, or equivalent in terms of dairy foods;
- energy and protein – include the one extra pint of semi-skimmed milk above and continue with the extra sandwich advised in pregnancy;
- vitamin A and C – continue to incorporate extra citrus fruit or fruit juice and extra vitamin A rich (generally orange/yellow coloured) fruit or vegetables into the diet, in addition to the two above recommendations;
- folate – encourage folate-rich foods;
- vitamin D – expose arms, face and legs to sunlight daily, during summer months.
- 'dietary fibre' – incorporate fruit, vegetables, and high fibre starchy foods;
- fluid should be advised as in pregnancy to prevent constipation.

4. Those women who have had a previous low birthweight infant should be targeted for preconceptional nutrition advice whilst still receiving postnatal care.
5. Every opportunity should be taken to advise those women who are underweight about how to achieve a 'normal' weight for both current and future pregnancies.
6. The Department of Health food safety recommendations (DoH 1992) should be addressed in combination with dietary advice.
7. More research is needed to explore nutrition during pregnancy and lactation.

■ **Practice check**

● Are mothers' dietary habits and use of nutritional supplements assessed in your area?
● What advice is given in your area on nutrition preconceptionally, and during pregnancy and lactation?
● What advice is given in your area on food safety during pregnancy?
● Do you take every available opportunity to promote a healthy, safe diet?

□ **Acknowledgments**

In compiling this chapter, the authors are grateful for the support of Hilary Warwick, Nutrition and Dietetic Services Manager, and Alison Dunnachie, Chief Dietitian, at Southampton General Hospital.

■ **References**

Abrams BF, Berman CA 1993 Nutrition during pregnancy and lactation. Primary Care 20(3): 585–97
Barker DJP, ed. 1992 Fetal and infant origins of adult disease. British Medical Journal, London
Barker DJP, Osmond C, Simmonds SJ, Wield GA 1993 The relation of small head circumference and thinness at birth to death from cardiovascular disease in adult life. British Medical Journal 306: 422–6
Bates CJ, Cowen TD, Tsuchiya H 1988 Growth, ascorbic acid and iron contents of tissues of young guinea-pigs whose dams received high or low levels of dietary ascorbic acid or Fe during pregnancy and suckling. British Journal of Nutrition 60: 487–97
Beyers N, Odendaal H, Hough F 1986 Vitamin D and mineral metabolism in normal pregnancy and in the normal foetus. South African Medical Journal 70: 549–53
Bhowmick S, Johnson R, Rettig R 1991 Call for clarification of vitamin D recommendations. Letter. American Journal of Diseases in Childhood 145(2): 127–30
British Dietetic Association 1993 Preconceptional nutrition: draft Position Paper. BDA, London
Bouillon R, Van Assche FA, Van Baelen H, Heyns W, De Moor P 1981 Influence of the vitamin D-binding protein on the serum concentration of 1,25-dihydroxyvitamin D3. Journal of Clinical Investigation 61: 589–96

Butte NF, Garza C, Stuff JE, Smith EO, Nichols BL 1984 Effect of maternal diet and body composition on lactational performance. American Journal of Clinical Nutrition 39: 296–306

Byerley LO, Kirksey A 1985 Effects of different levels of vitamin C intake on the vitamin C concentration in human milk and the vitamin C intakes of breast-fed infants. American Journal of Clinical Nutrition 41: 665–71

Carr P, Rothburn M 1989 Listeriosis in midwifery. Nursing Times 85(18): 73–4

Caird, L 1989 Listeriosis in pregnancy. Letter. Lancet 1: 322

Childrens' Nutrition Research Centre 1991 European Journal of Clinical Nutrition 45: 227–42

Cockburn F, Belton NR, Purvis RJ 1980 Maternal vitamin D intake and mineral metabolism in mothers and their newborn infants. British Medical Journal 281: 11–14

Committee on Iron Deficiency 1968 Iron deficiency in the United States. Journal of the American Medical Association 203: 407–12

Coward WA, Paul AA, Prentice AM 1984 The impact of malnutrition on human lactation: observations from community studies. Federal Proceedings 43(9): 296–306

Delvin E, Salle M, Glorieux F, Adeleine P, David M 1986 Vitamin D supplementation during pregnancy; effect on neonatal calcium homeostasis. Journal of Paediatrics 109(2): 328–33

Department of Health 1988 Salmonella and raw eggs. DoH, London

Department of Health 1989 Listeriosis and food. Letter. DoH, London

Department of Health 1990 Women cautioned: watch your vitamin A intake. DoH, London

Department of Health 1991 Dietary Reference Values for food energy and nutrients for the United Kingdom. Report of the Panel on Dietary Reference Values of the Committee on Medical Aspects of Food Policy. Report on Health and Social Subjects No 41. HMSO, London

Department of Health 1992 While you are pregnant: safe eating and how to avoid infection from food and animals. DoH, London

Department of Health 1993 Vitamin A and pregnancy. Letter. DoH, London

Doyle W, Crawford MA, Wynn AHA, Wynn SW 1989 Maternal nutrient intake and birthweight. Journal of Human Nutrition and Dietetics 2: 415–22

Doyle W, Crawford MA, Wynn AHA, Wynn SW 1990 The association between maternal diet and birth dimensions. Journal of Nutritional Medicine 1: 9–17

Durnin JVGA 1991 Energy requirements of pregnancy. Acta Paediatrica Scandanavica 373: 33–42

Expert Advisory Group on Folic Acid 1992 Folic acid and the prevention of neural tube defects. DoH, London

FAO/WHO/UNU 1985 Energy and protein requirements. Report of a joint expert consultation. WHO Technical Rep. Ser. No. 724. WHO, Geneva

Forsum E, Lonnerdahl B 1980 Effect of protein intake on protein and nitrogen composition of breast milk. American Journal of Clinical Nutrition 33: 1809–13

Ganguly C, Mukherjee KL 1988 Relationship between maternal serum vitamin A and vitamin A status of the corresponding fetuses. Journal of Tropical Paediatrics 34: 313–15

Gilbert RJ, Miller KL, Roberts D 1989 Listeria monocytogenes and chilled foods. Lancet 1: 383–4

Giroud A 1973 Nutritional requirements of the embryo. World Reviews of Nutrition and Dietetics 18: 195–262

Greer F, Tsang R, Searcy J, Levin R, Steichen J 1982 Mineral homeostasis during lactation – relationship to serum 1,25-dihydroxyvitamin D, 25-hydroxyvitamin D, parathyroid hormone and calcitonin. American Journal Clinical Nutrition 38: 431–7

Gregory J, Foster K, Tyler H, Wiseman M 1990 The dietary and nutritional survey of British adults. HMSO, London

Health Education Authority 1994 New pregnancy book. HEA, London

Heaney R, Skillman T 1971 Calcium metabolism in normal human pregnancy. Journal of Human Endocrinology and Metabolism 33: 661–70

Hibbard E, Smithells R 1965 Folic acid metabolism and human embryopathy. Lancet 1: 1254

Hytten FE, Leitch I 1971 The physiology of human pregnancy. Blackwell Scientific Publications, Oxford: 163–229

Hytten FE 1983 Nutritional physiology during pregnancy. In Campbell DM, Gillmer MDG (eds) Nutrition in pregnancy. Royal College of Obstetricians and Gynaecologists, London

Kent N, Price I, Gutteridge D, Rosman R, Smith M, Allen J, Hickling C, Blakeman S 1991 The efficiency of intestinal calcium absorption is increased in late pregnancy but not in established lactation. Calcified Tissue International 48: 293–5

Kramer M 1987 Determinants of low birthweight: Methodological assessment and meta-analysis. Bulletin of the WHO 65(5): 663–737

Lamont RJ, Postlethwaite R 1986 Carriage of *Listeria monocytogenes* and related species in pregnant and non-pregnant women in Aberdeen, Scotland. Journal of Infection 13: 187–93

Laurence KM, James N, Miller N, Tennant G, Campbell H 1981 Double blind randomised controlled trial of folate treatment before conception to prevent recurrence of NTD. British Medical Journal 1282: 1509–11

Misra R, Anderson D 1990 Providing the foetus with calcium. British Medical Journal 300: 1220–21

Montgomery E 1993 Iron and vitamin supplementation during pregnancy. In Alexander J, Levy V, Roch S (eds) Midwifery practice: a research based approach, vol. 4. Macmillan, Basingstoke

National Research Council, Food & Nutrition Board 1989 Recommendations of dietary allowances. National Academy Press, Washington DC

Nelson M 1990 Vitamin A, liver consumption, and risk of birth defects. British Medical Journal 301: 1176

Niswander KR, Gordon M 1972 The women and their pregnancies. US Department of Health, Education and Welfare, Washington DC

Obstetrics Committee 1993 Vitamin A supplementation during pregnancy. International Journal of Gynaecology and Obstetrics 40: 175

Office of Population Censuses and Surveys 1988 Congenital malformation statistics 1981–85: notifications England and Wales. Series MB3 No. 2 HMSO, London

Pini PN, Gilbert RJ 1988 The occurrence in the UK of Listeria species in raw chickens and soft cheeses. International Journal of Food Microbiology 6: 317–26

Purdie DW 1989 Bone mineral metabolism and reproduction. Contemporary Reviews in Obstetrics and Gynaecology 1: 214–21

Quentin C, Thibaut MC, Horovitz J, Bebear C 1990 Multiresistant strain of Listeria monocytogenes in septic abortion. Letter. Lancet 336: 375

Rosa FW, Wilk AL, Kelsey FO 1986 Teratogen update: vitamin A congeners. Teratology 33: 355–64

Sanchez-Poso A, Lopez-Morales J, Ixquierdo A, Gil A 1987 Protein composition of human milk in relation to mother's weight and socio-economic status. Human Nutrition: Clinical Nutrition 41C: 115–25

Schiffman RL, Tejani N, Verma U, McNerney R 1989 Effect of dietary protein on glomerular filtration rate in pregnancy. Obstetrics and Gynaecology 73(1): 47–51

Schonberg K (Chairman) 1989 Adolescent pregnancy. A statement from the American Academy of Pediatrics Committee on Adolescence. Pediatrics 83(1): 132–3

Smithells R, Nevin N, Seller M, Sheppard S, Harris R, Read A *et al* 1983 Further experience of vitamin supplementation for prevention of NTD recurrences. Lancet 1: 1027–31

Sulaiman ND 1988 Alcohol consumption in Dundee primigravidas and its effects on outcome of pregnancy. British Medical Journal 296: 1500–3

Svanberg B, Arvidsson B, Bjorn-Rasmussen E, Hallberg L, Rossander L, Swolin B 1975 Dietary iron absorption in pregnancy: a longitudinal study with repeated measurements of non-haem iron absorption from the whole diet. Acta Obstetrica et Gynaecologia Scandinavica 48 (supp): 43–68

Strode MA, Dewey KG, Lonnerdal B 1986 Effects of short-term caloric restriction on lactational performance of well-nourished women. Acta Paediatrica Scandanavica 75: 222–9

Teratology Society 1975 Recommendations for vitamin A use during pregnancy. Teratology 35: 269–75

The MRC Vitamin Study Group 1991 Prevention of neural tube defects: results of the Medical Research Council Vitamin Study. Lancet 2: 131–7

Thomas MR, Irving CS, Reeds PJ, Malphus EW, Wong WW, Boutton TW, Klein PD 1991 Lysine and protein metabolism in the young lactating woman. European Journal of Clinical Nutrition 45(5): 227–42

Van der Spuy AM, Steer PJ, Mccusker M, Steele SJ, Jacobs HS 1988 Outcome of pregnancy in underweight women after spontaneous and induced ovulation. British Medical Journal 296: 962–5

Verkerk PH, van Noord-Zaadstar BM, Florey CV, de Jonge GA, Verloove-Vanhorick SP 1993 The effect of moderate maternal alcohol consumption on birth weight and gestational age in a low risk population. Early Human Development 32: 121–9

Vuori E 1979 Intake of copper, iron, manganese and zinc by healthy, exclusively breast-fed infants during the first 3 months of life. British Journal of Nutrition 42: 407–11

Winick M, Rosso P 1975 Malnutrition and central nervous system development. In Prescott JW, Read NA, Coursin D (eds). Brain function and malnutrition: neuropsychogical methods of assessment. John Wiley, New York

Whitehead RG 1983 Dietary supplementation of lactating Gambian women: effect on breast milk volume and quality. Journal of Human Nutrition and Clinical Nutrition 37C: 53–64

Whittaker PG, Lind T, Williams JG 1991 Iron absorption during normal human pregnancy: a study using stable isotopes. British Journal of Nutrition 65: 457–63

Wilson S, Retallack R, Kent J, Worth G, Gutteridge D 1990 Serum free 1,25-dihydroxyvitamin D and the free 1,25-dihydroxyvitamin D index during a longitudinal study of human pregnancy and lactation. Clinical Endocrinology 32: 613–22

Worthington-Roberts B, Rodwell-Williams S 1989 Nutrition in pregnancy and lactation. Times Mirror/Mosby, St Louis

Wynn A, Wynn M 1990 The need for nutritional assessment in the treatment of the infertile patient. Journal of Nutritional Medicine 1: 315–24

Wynn AHA, Crawford MA, Doyle W, Wynn SW 1991 Nutrition of women in anticipation of pregnancy. Nutrition and Health 7: 69–88

■ Suggested further reading

Department of Health 1991 Dietary Reference Values for food energy and nutrients for the United Kingdom. Report of the Panel on Dietary Reference Values of the Committee on Medical Aspects of Food Policy. Report on Health and Social Subjects No. 41. HMSO, London

Department of Health 1992 While you are pregnant: safe eating and how to avoid infection from food and animals. DoH, London

Expert Advisory Group on Folic Acid 1992 Folic acid and the prevention of neural tube defects. DoH, London

Health Education Authority 1993 The new pregnancy book. HEA, London
Thomas B 1994 Manual of dietetic practice, 2nd edn. Blackwell Scientific Publications, Oxford
Truswell S 1992 ABC of nutrition. British Medical Journal, London

Chapter 2

Midwifery care during the first stage of labour

Rosaline Steele

> The woman must be the focus of maternity care. She should be able to feel that she is in control of what is happening to her and be able to make decisions about her care, based on her needs, having discussed matters fully with the professionals involved
>
> Expert Maternity Group 1993:9

This statement, from the report 'Changing childbirth', has been highlighted as 'the first principle of the maternity services'. This is a reaffirmation of the belief held by women and many midwives, that the process of pregnancy and childbearing belong to the woman, and that midwives and other professionals are partners in the process, not 'chief executives'. As a woman approaches childbirth, she needs to feel that the choices she has made about the conduct of her labour and delivery will be respected. In order for midwives to facilitate the needs of a woman during labour, the decisions she has made about her care should be thoroughly discussed and planned with her. This approach would mean that midwives would have to review their current practice, particularly as it relates to the care of women during the first stage of labour.

> The part which the midwife plays in maternity care should make full use of all her skills and knowledge, and reflect the full role for which she has been trained.
>
> Expert Maternity Group 1993: 39

The focus of this chapter will be on the changes which may be needed in the practice of some midwives in their approach to caring for women during the first stage of labour, changes which will facilitate 'woman focused' care and which will move care away from some of the rituals which have become associated with caring for women in labour. Immobilisation and starvation are but two of these rituals.

The most effective way in which changes in practice could be brought about is through the utilisation of research findings and reflection on practice which may generate further areas for research. The work of Romney (1980) and Romney and Gordon (1981) on enemas and perineal shaving are examples of how the utilisation of research can change practice. However, change in practice may often be slow; Drayton (1990) indicates that many maternity units were still giving women enemas as part of the admission procedure as late as 1989. Change in practice as a result of research should occur more rapidly in the future as more midwives are involved in the initiation and evaluation of research.

It must be acknowledged that not all women will want or be able to have midwife only care. This may be for a variety of reasons, for example, the woman's choice or a complication of pregnancy or labour. Nevertheless whether the midwife is the lead professional or not, the care she gives a woman should be individual to her needs.

The issues which will be discussed include the organisation and planning of care, the place of birth, stress and the birth environment, nutrition and fluids during labour and the importance of support in labour.

■ It is assumed that you are already aware of the following:

- The physiology of normal labour;
- The anatomy of the female genital tract;
- The recommendations of the Expert Maternity Group (1993) in their report, 'Changing childbirth'.

■ The organisation of care

□ Continuity of care

The view that women want to have continuity of care is well documented (Social Services Committee 1980; MSAC 1982; HC

Health Committee 1992; Expert Maternity Group 1993). There-fore, the organisation of midwifery care must be such that it allows for this continuity. The midwife will need to move away from the artificial barriers which have been erected between hospital and community. Practitioners should have their own caseloads and take responsibility for the woman throughout her pregnancy (Page 1993). A seamless pattern of care must be the norm if women are to be able to choose who they would like to care for them, how the care should be conducted and where they would like to have their babies.

A number of initiatives have been taken by practitioners and consumers in many parts of the UK to improve the quality of the childbirth experience. Many of these initiatives are related to the organisation of midwifery care using a team approach. However, Wraight *et al* (1993) found that there was no clear definition of what was meant by 'team midwifery'. They placed the information elicited from the managers on the definitions of teams into ten categories and three key phrases emerged:

- Team midwifery involves total care;
- Team midwifery involves recognised caseloads;
- Team midwifery involves continuity of care.

None of the units sampled in the study indicated that the women had the opportunity to choose their carer/carers or how they would like their care conducted.

The 'Know your midwife' (KYM) scheme was evaluated by a study (Flint & Poulengeris 1987) designed to test whether it was possible for a small group of midwives to give total care to a group of women with the purpose of offering continuity of care. While they were in labour, the women in this group normally had a midwife with them who they had been able to get to know during their pregnancy. The women's satisfaction with the scheme was measured through self-administered questionnaires which were distributed at 37 weeks of pregnancy, two days postnatally and six weeks postnatally. Forty-two per cent of the women who were delivered by a midwife who was known to them described their labour as a positive experience. Only 24 per cent of the women who did not know the midwives delivering their babies described the experience as positive.

Klein *et al* (1983) carried out a retrospective study which compared the care of low risk women in a shared care (consult-ant) system and an integrated general practitioner (GP) unit system. The organisation of the midwifery staff in the GP unit system had the same features as the KYM scheme. There were no significant differences in the social or obstetric characteristics of the women in the study, which featured nulliparous and multiparous subjects. The women in the GP unit had fewer inductions, used less analgesia and had fewer forceps deliveries. The findings are statistically significant in the multiparous group; 27 per cent of the women in that group booked for shared care had their labour induced while the figure was 10 per cent for the GP unit booked women. The figures for forceps deliveries were 8 per cent for the shared care group and 1 per cent for the GP unit booked women.

Currell, a midwife, undertook a comparative study of shared care, GP unit care and home delivery care in 1985. The study sought to test the hypothesis that the organisational patterns of midwifery care would be found along a continuum with continuity of care at one end and fragmented care at the other. Currell (1990) found fragmentation of care in all groups except for a small proportion of women who had a home delivery, and did not observe any statistically significant differences between the groups in the ways that women perceived the quality of communication during pregnancy or support during labour. She concludes, 'Care that is ineffective, inappropriate, unacceptable, or simply wrong, can be of no value even if it is given under the umbrella of "continuity"' (Currell 1990).

The beneficial findings of the KYM scheme have encouraged many providers of midwifery care to review their organisation of care and several initiatives have been developed which are more woman-centred. These initiatives were mainly based on the team approach to midwifery care, which according to the evidence of Wraight and colleagues (1993) has had variable success. The failure of team midwifery schemes was mainly due to the implementation process; for example, in some of the units sampled there was little consultation with staff prior to the introduction of teams, therefore the process of change was slower, and the staffing levels needed by the teams to care effectively for women were not identified. This in the view of the midwives reduced the choices about care that the woman could make (Wraight *et al* 1993).

If the targets set by the Expert Maternity Group (1993) are to be met in the required time, workable woman-centred schemes need to be developed. The midwives who manage the maternity services have the challenge of leading the change in philosophy which will be needed if the service is to offer continuity of care. Hauxwell and Tanner (1994) found that to achieve continuity of care they had to facilitate a large culture shift, which resulted in the total integration of the hospital and community midwifery services. The women in their care now have a named midwife with whom they can plan their care.

☐ **Planning care**

> Women should have the opportunity to discuss their plans
> for labour and birth. Their decisions should be recorded
> in their birth plans and incorporated into their case
> notes . . .
>
> Expert Maternity Group 1993: 31

Respect for a woman's individual needs, and her involvement in decisions about her care is essential throughout pregnancy, but is crucial during labour. To ensure that the woman's individual needs and wishes are known, a plan of care should be developed by the woman and the midwife. This plan of care, which should include the start of a birth plan (Kitzinger 1987), should begin ideally at the time of the antenatal booking interview. Methven (1989) highlighted the problem of the booking interview being confined to a series of pre-printed questions which are part of the case notes. The information obtained was often not a sound enough foundation on which to plan a woman's care with her. During her research on individualised care in midwifery, Bryar (1991) found that even when care plans were developed they were rarely referred to while care was being implemented. Identified problems and future plans were usually recorded after the woman had been seen.

In order to plan with a woman the care she wants, midwives need to listen to what she is saying. 'Listening refers to the process of hearing what the client is saying' (Burnard 1990: 98). Listening is central to effective communication. Kirkham (1983) found that during admission in labour, a woman would give lengthy descriptions in answer to questions about the onset of labour. As the form being completed by the midwife did not require a lengthy answer, the response from the midwife was usually brief. This resulted in the woman's responses becoming shorter thereby causing a breakdown in communication between the woman and the midwife. The woman then found it difficult to seek information about the progress of her labour because she felt inhibited about asking questions. Read and Garcia (1989) indicate that very often women find it difficult to ask questions of professionals unless they are encouraged to do so.

Midwives with developed listening skills should be able to hear what the woman is really saying, and should encourage her to ask questions, thereby developing a conduit for the exchange of information. Kirkham (1993) argues that if the questions women ask are answered immediately and clearly, then they will feel free to ask further questions. This exchange should facilitate the development of a plan of care. However, in order to be able to participate in planning her care a woman must have information on which to base her choices.

☐ **Choice**

> Unless women are given sufficient balanced non judgemental and appropriate information at each stage of the maternity process they are unlikely to feel able to make informed choices about their care.
> (HC Health Committee 1992)

Choices are only as good as the information on which they are based (Mander 1993). The information that women receive may come from the media, the experience of friends or relations and from general literature. Information given to the woman by the midwife should be based on well researched sources so that the woman has as many facts as possible at her disposal to enable her to make decisions about her care. A study by Green and colleagues (1990) suggested that information which enabled women to make decisions and feel in control, not only enhanced their experience of birth but was beneficial to their emotional wellbeing following delivery. However, midwives need to be conscious of the factors which could affect the quality of information that they give women. For example, Kirkham (1989) states that from her research she found that a woman's social class governed the amount and type of information she received from the midwife. Women in the higher social groups received more information from midwives in response to their questions and often had information volunteered to them. However, women from the lower social groups did not have the same skill at eliciting information from midwives and had to ask repeated questions as the midwives did not volunteer extra information. These latter women were often viewed as disruptive because they did not conform to the midwife's view of the 'good patient,' those being the ones who did not pose a threat to the authority of the midwives, by asking too many questions.

■ The place of birth

> Purchasers should as part of their strategic plan, review the
> current choices available to women regarding the place of
> birth. Following consultation, these should be developed as
> appropriate for their locality and ensure that home birth is
> a real option for women who may wish to have it; and
> ensure that women receive information about the full
> range of options for place of birth available in her locality.
>
> Expert Maternity Group 1993: 25

As midwives help women to make decisions about where they
would like to have their babies, thought should not only be given
to the objectives of 'Changing childbirth' (Expert Maternity Group
1993) but also to the research evidence relating to the place of
birth.

In many areas of the UK the policy on place of birth is still
based on the belief that hospital is the safest place to give birth
and that the reduction in the perinatal mortality rate has been
due to increase in the number of hospital births (Campbell 1990).
This belief was built upon the recommendations of the Peel report (DHSS 1970), one of the key recommendations of which
was that: 'the resources of modern medicine' should be available to all mothers and babies, and to this end there should be
sufficient resources for every mother in the country to have a
hospital delivery. The committee did not produce any evidence
to support the view that hospital confinement was always safer,
but did draw attention to the reduction in the perinatal mortality rate and the rise in hospital confinements. In their review
'Where to be born?', Campbell and Macfarlane (1987) argue
that the debate which the report generated was not always supported by reliable statistical and epidemiological information. The
assumption that hospital delivery is safer for all women was chal-
lenged by Tew (1987), whose analysis of the published maternal
and perinatal mortality data suggested that death rates for mother
and fetus were higher in hospital than in the home. Tew's analysis
was carried out for comparable groups.

The debate about the place of birth is often conducted as if
there are only two places in which women can give birth, at
home or in hospital (Campbell & Macfarlane 1987). A study by
Taylor (1986) found that women wanted care other than that
available in consultant obstetric units. General practitioner units
are reducing in number and this has the effect of reducing the
choice of place of birth available to women (Campbell *et al* 1991).
Bryce *et al* (1990) and Sangala *et al* (1990) seemed to suggest

that the care offered by GP units was less safe than that available in consultant obstetric units, although substantial evidence to the contrary exists (Campbell & Macfarlane 1987; Prentice & Walton 1989). While few studies have been undertaken to measure morbidity in mothers and babies (Campbell *et al* 1991), a study which compared similar groups of low risk women who delivered under the care of GPs and consultant obstetricians found that morbidity was higher in those who had had consultant care (Klein *et al* 1983). Low risk women who were in the comparative studies of home or hospital births demonstrated similar results, that is higher morbidity in the births which took place in hospital (Mehl 1978; Shearer 1985). Furthermore, a second (prospective) study by Klein and colleagues (1985) did not find any significant evidence to support the view that morbidity was higher under consultant care.

Wherever women choose to have their babies, midwives will be providing most if not all of the care, therefore, it is vital that the midwife's practice is researched based. This approach should enable the woman and midwife to feel confident about the process in whatever setting the birth takes place.

■ Care in labour

□ Stress and the birth environment

A woman in labour will experience a variety of new sensations (Kitzinger 1987), particularly if it is her first delivery. Garforth and Garcia (1989) identified conflicting emotions such as excitement, anxiety, fear and apprehension which are experienced by women as they enter labour. If the midwife caring for the woman is known to her, then some of some of the anxiety she may experience is reduced (Flint 1991). The environment in which the labour takes place can have a significant effect on the amount of fear and anxiety experienced by the woman. Kirkham (1989) found during her study on information giving in labour, that women who laboured in their own homes, felt confident about taking clinical decisions about their labours because it was 'their territory'. The relationship between the midwife and the woman was such that they were more like colleagues taking decisions together about the progress of labour.

When a woman is admitted to hospital in labour, regardless of how homely the room is made to look, she may still feel alienated by the environment. For example, the simple act of placing a name band on her wrist reduces her autonomy (Hall 1993). Other activities, such as asking the woman to undress on admission, or performing a vaginal examination when there is a lack of privacy (Flint 1984; Garforth & Garcia 1989) would further give the feeling of loss of control.

Jowitt (1993) argues that situations which cause us to feel that we cannot influence our environment and the people within it will result in our stress levels being raised. She further states that in hospital, where the woman cannot control the environment, she is more likely to experience high levels of stress. Jowitt cites Bohus and de Kloet (1979) who believe that beta-endorphin secretion, which is raised during stress, has both physiological and psychological effects – enhancing memory in addition to suppressing smooth muscle. If women are stressed by their environment, labour could be prolonged because of the reduced contractility of the uterus (Zuspan 1962; Lederman *et al* 1985).

From her study of women's birth experience, Simkin (1991; 1992) formed the view that when women were denied control of their birth experience, their memory of the event was very often distressing. As discussed above, lack of control is a stressor. Furthermore, if beta-endorphins (which are produced in greater amounts in response to stress) enhance memory, then the woman will carry the negative experience with her for life. It would seem eminently sensible for midwives always to be aware not only of the joy they can help women to experience around the time of birth and after, but also the long term psychological damage that can occur if women are not empowered to take control of their birth experience.

☐ **Nutrition and fluids in labour**

Johnson and colleagues (1989) state that many aspects of care during labour and childbirth lead to keen discussion. For example, a controversial topic is whether or not women should have free access to food and drink. Grant's (1990) comprehensive chapter on nutrition and fluids in labour (in Volume 2 of this series) is central to the debate on oral fluids and nutrition in labour.

In the mid 1980s, a survey of labour ward policies in England (Garcia *et al* 1986) revealed that over a third of the consultant maternity units discouraged oral fluids and foods during labour. Many of these policies were developed in response to the high maternal death rate associated with general anaesthesia. These deaths were mainly attributed to the aspiration of gastric contents, which resulted in a syndrome classically described by Mendelson (1946) and which now bears his name.

The aspiration of gastric contents is now a very small contributor to the number of maternal deaths. In the most recent report on the Confidential Enquiries into Maternal Deaths 1988–90 (DoH 1994), there were four direct maternal deaths associated with anaesthesia in the UK, only two of which were attributed to the aspiration of gastric contents.

The prevention of mortality and morbidity related to pregnancy and childbearing is essential, and the death of one woman during this period is a death too many. However, it is necessary to review current practices so as to facilitate the development of appropriate care policies.

The policy of restricting diet and fluids in labour which may be the correct management for women with a substantial chance of needing general anaesthesia is now widespread (Johnson *et al* 1989). Approximately 75 per cent of women in England and Wales are delivered by a midwife who is the most senior person present (Robinson *et al* 1983), those women therefore would not usually need a general anaesthetic. It would seem that the practice of restricting food and fluids to *all* women in labour reduces considerably the woman's choice and the opportunity for midwives to use their clinical judgement as they care for women. Robinson (1989) identified that the midwife's freedom to make clinical decisions about the basic care of women in labour had to large extent been curtailed. This in her view was largely due to obstetric unit policies.

In 1990, the first of four 'Recommendations for clinical practice' made by Judith Grant in the light of the research evidence then available, was:

> When it is considered that the client in labour has no risk factors for requiring instrumental delivery or general anaesthesia, she should be allowed to eat a light diet and drink as she requires. A light diet should contain foods which are easily absorbed by the stomach. It will therefore be very low in fats and roughage and only small amounts should be eaten at one time.
>
> Grant 1990: 66

As midwives review their practice relating to the offering of fluids and food to labouring women, attention should be paid to the likely physiological and psychological effects of restricting a woman's diet in labour. Grant (1990) emphasises the normality of eating and drinking and suggests that being able to perform these activities of everyday living may increase the woman's feeling of wellbeing and reduce her stress level. In addition, the withholding of food may also have very unpleasant side-effects from the action of an empty stomach, contracting with increasing intensity (Hinchliff & Montague 1989). Women who will already be experiencing the pain of uterine contractions should not be subjected to further discomfort.

An American study (Ludka 1987) cited and discussed fully by Grant (1990:59) suggests that the withholding of food and drink from labouring women results in increased need for augmentation of labour, instrumental delivery, caesarean section and neonatal intensive care.

A small study conducted by a midwife, Angela Flanagan, and an anaesthetist, Kieran Fitzpatrick, looked at the outcomes of babies and the length of labour of women who ate and drank during labour (Flanagan 1992). Forty women in labour were encouraged to eat foods such as toast, eggs, yoghurt, ice cream, jellies and fresh fruit. A control group of 22 women had the usual tea and toast in early labour and sips of water thereafter. The results of the study showed that women in the first group required less pain relief, less chemical stimulation of the uterus and the length of labour was reduced. The Apgar scores of the babies of the women in the first group were higher than those in the control group. As a result of the study the restriction on oral intake during labour in the Jubilee Maternity Unit is more liberal. This study is being replicated using a larger sample.

The reader is referred to Grant (1990:60–61) for a discussion of ketonuria in labour in the context of whether or not women in labour should be permitted oral refreshment. She claims that 'The presence of small amounts of ketones in the urine can be interpreted as being a normal physiological occurrence'.

The reduction of food and drink in labour may result in ketosis and dehydration (Johnson *et al* 1989; Grant 1990). The administration of an intravenous infusion to prevent and treat ketosis and dehydration should not be regarded as completely safe. Grant's 'Recommendation for clinical practice' in the light of the research evidence available in 1990 was:

> When intravenous fluids are administered, an accurate
> fluid balance record must be maintained. The
> administration rate should not exceed 1.5 ml/kg/hour, nor
> should the fluid contain more than 10 g of Dextrose per
> hour. Iso-osmotic fluids such as Dextrose-saline or
> Hartmann's solution should be used.
>
> Grant 1990: 67

Swift (1991) argues that the act of setting up an intravenous infusion on a woman in normal labour may have a cascade of unwanted outcomes, including the possibility of iatrogenic infection from the siting of a cannula and the reduction of mobility which may cause the woman to feel she is no longer in control of her labour. Restriction of mobility was identified by Simkin (1986) as being seen as highly stressful by 25 per cent of subjects and high levels of stress and anxiety have themselves been associated with a reduction in uterine activity (Lederman *et al* 1978; 1985).

As midwives, we have an obligation to ensure that all of the care being offered to our clients is based on well researched, contemporary information. It could be argued that the withholding of food and fluids from women in normal labour does not reflect the research evidence. Midwives should examine this evidence and then decide whether the practices currently in use in their unit should remain unchallenged.

■ Support during childbirth

So far in this chapter the focus has been on Choice, Continuity and Change. Choice for the woman in the selection of her carers and the place of birth, continuity of care so that her choice is meaningful and the change in the midwife's practice which may be necessary if the needs of the woman are to be met. These are three Cs which underpinned the Consensus Conference on Maternity Care, held in London on the 4–5th March, 1993. There are another three Cs which will be introduced at this stage, not only because of their relevance to the care of a woman during the first stage of labour, but because together they embody the essence of support for women during childbirth. They are Comfort, Confidence and Companionship.

□ 'With woman'

As the place of birth has moved from the home into hospital, the emotional support which was provided by the woman's family and friends, and a midwife who was known to her, is no longer available (Bowes 1992). The technology and intervention which is a feature of many labour wards, leave women feeling vulnerable and dissatisfied with their birth experience (Brown & Lumley 1994).

In discussing support in labour it is not only the emotional aspect which is under consideration but physical support and advocacy. Advocacy on the part of the midwife involves ensuring that the woman's stated plans for her labour are not disrupted because of labour ward procedures. Comfort, confidence and companionship may also come from a variety of other sources. For the purposes of this chapter three types of supporters will be considered, the woman's partner, other individuals such as birth attendants, and finally the midwife.

☐ Support from the woman's partner

In the last 20 years women's male partners have played a significant role in giving support during labour, particularly in the hospital setting. Keirse *et al* (1989) offer two reasons for the entrance of male partners into the labour ward. The first of these is the move by women to de-medicalise the birth experience and the inclusion of the father of the baby at a crucial time in the event as a part of that process. The partners would also be able to reinforce coping techniques for labour which had been learnt in the antenatal period and act as an advocate if an attempt was made to disrupt these techniques. The second reason is that partners would be able to give the psychological support which was not available from the otherwise busy staff. Niven (1985) suggests that some partners provide essential psychological and physical support during labour. Activities such as back rubbing and active encouragement with breathing techniques were viewed by the women in labour as particularly helpful (Niven 1985).

Summersgill (1993) offers other reasons for the increased presence of male partners in the labour ward. He argues that our culture does not have a mechanism through which the importance of the expectant father can be recognised, therefore, in order to gain some social recognition for their new position as fathers, they have developed the ritual known as couvade. Examples of this include the acquisition of technical knowledge by the fathers which they use to help their partners make decisions about labour options – obtaining information which can be used by them to assist their partner in decisions about pain relief in labour.

Lewis (1986) states that fathers are often the central source for the transmission of information, particularly when the woman had analgesia and was in the active phase of labour. Although Lewis found that men were eager to support their partners during labour, some were very apprehensive but were persuaded to attend by family members and their partners.

Niven (1985) found from her research on the presence of a chosen birth companion and the woman's level of pain in labour, that there was no significant difference in the amount of pain experienced by women who did not have their partner with her, as compared those whose partner was present. She found, however, that women who positively welcomed the presence of their partner had lower levels of labour pain compared to all other subjects. She concluded that it was not just the presence of the partner but the woman's feelings about his presence that could make a difference.

A study of Asian women's experience of childbirth in East London (Woolet & Dosanjh-Matwala 1990) found that the majority of women were pleased to have their husbands present at birth and considered their support important. Only 13 of the 32 women interviewed had been born in the UK. From the study it did not appear that female members of the family were central to labour support. They concluded that the loosening of traditional family ties accounted for the more central role now being taken by husbands in labour. Odent (1984) suggests a negative effect on the progress of a woman's labour if there is tension between the couple, he argues that the woman's labour is likely to be prolonged and that the practical and emotional support may difficult to provide or to accept. Although there is no current evidence which could help to evaluate whether the support of a woman's male partner in labour makes a difference to its outcome, in the opinion of the author the emotional and practical benefit that most women seem to gain from the support of their partner is evident.

□ **Support from others**

Sosa *et al* (1980) and Klaus *et al* (1986) demonstrated from their two studies done in Guatemala the benefit of the continuous presence of a supportive companion in labour. The companion used was a *doula*, an experienced woman who does not provide midwifery care but guides and supports new mothers in child care. The mothers in the study were first introduced to their doula when they were in labour. In their 1986 study Klaus and Colleagues demonstrated statistically significant differences in the labour outcomes of women who were supported by a doula. Seventeen per cent of the women who were not supported were delivered by a caesarean section, while only 7 per cent of the supported group were delivered in that way. Augmentation of labour with oxytocin was needed by 13 per cent of the control group, but only 7 per cent of the experimental group needed this intervention.

To identify whether similar results could be obtained in a more technological environment, Kennell and colleagues (1991) undertook a randomised controlled trial which examined the medical effects of support during labour. The study was conducted in an American public hospital providing care for a low income black, white and Hispanic population. The 412 women in the study were randomly allocated, 212 to the support group (where a doula was assigned to each woman to give continuous support), and 200 to the observed group (the group was monitored by an inconspicuous observer). A further group, a control group, was made up of women who were admitted to the hospital on days that doulas were already assigned to women. The 204 women in this group had to meet the same criteria as the other two groups.

The doulas had a three week training period to enable them to become familiar with the hospital policies and labour procedures. The result of the study showed that, in the supported group, the caesarean section rate was 8 per cent, in the observed group it was 13 per cent, and in the control group it was 18 per cent. Approximately 11 per cent of the babies from the supported group remained in hospital for medical reasons, this figure was 17 per cent for the observed group and 24 per cent for the control group. The positive outcomes from the observed group led the researchers to surmise that the continuous presence of the observer may have acted as a source of comfort to the woman.

If properly implemented, the role of the midwife in the UK negates the need for a doula. Taylor (1991) argues that to encourage the use of birth attendants is to encourage further fragmentation of maternity care. However, an article by James (1990) on her work as a birth attendant in England in which she acted as a 'shield' for women in labour should encourage midwives to question why some women might find this support necessary.

☐ **Midwife's support**

> I see the midwife as the supporter and sometimes therefore the defender of the woman she cares for in labour, but to achieve this we must really concentrate on the woman and her needs.
>
> Kirkham 1986: 40

Preparing for the birth To concentrate fully on a woman's needs the midwife should have gathered as much information as possible about the woman and her pregnancy prior to the start of labour. Ideally, the preparation of a birth plan by the woman and the midwife would have identified the key areas of support which will be needed during labour. Kitzinger (1987) defines a birth plan as 'a concise written statement' of wishes for childbirth and the days following birth. In this author's experience, however, some midwives are concerned that in the event of a complication of labour the woman's birth plan could exclude them from taking what in their professional judgement is the appropriate action. Dimond (1993) suggests that, when midwives are preparing birth plans with women, they should ensure that the women are aware that the plan is subject to the clinical situation and that the midwife may need to deviate from the plan should it be clinically necessary. Some women experience feelings of failure and disappointment when their birth does not go according to plan (Wolf 1990), and Swinnerton (1990) suggests that antenatal care and education should help women to avoid becoming obsessed with the perfect birth.

Pickrell and Marshall (1989) indicate that operative delivery (caesarean section or instrumental vaginal delivery) were as much as four times greater in women who prepared birth plans than those who did not. Smoleniec and James (1992) undertook a retrospective review of the case notes of 124 women with normal singleton pregnancies, 62 with birth plans and 62 without. Their aim was to test the hypothesis that having a birth plan for labour was associated with an increased risk of operative delivery. Their findings indicate that there was no significant difference in the operative delivery rate between the two groups 27 per cent of the birth plan group had operative deliveries (24 per cent operative vaginal and 3 per cent caesarean section). In the non-birth plan group, 32 per cent had operative deliveries (27 per cent operative vaginal and 5 per cent caesarean section).

Information giving Brown and Lumley (1994) surveyed 790 Australian women to ascertain their satisfaction with care in labour and birth. Their analysis showed that women were dissatisfied when insufficient information was given, when they were not offered the opportunity to make decisions about their care and when caregivers were unhelpful. A study by Fleissig (1993) on information giving by staff during labour found that during childbirth women wanted constant support and information about the progress of their labour.

The role of midwives in Britain puts them in a unique position to offer the type of support that women in labour appear to want. Midwives can assess the progress of a woman's labour, identify deviations from the norm and enable the woman to make decisions about what action should be taken. In spite of being in this unique role, Kirkham (1989) found that many midwives did not give women the information they needed, the midwives concerned reported that this was in most cases due to the constraints of hospital policies, inhibiting presence of senior staff and in some cases lack of experience. Kirkham argues that many of the problems associated with our communication with clients stems from the way in which care is organised. She states that the fragmented nature of care prevents practitioners from establishing adequate communication with women (Kirkham 1993). In her observation of midwives' information giving during labour, the same author found that many midwives gave women a large amount of information in a very short space of time. Much of the information dealt with procedure for labour, so women did not often have an opportunity to discuss their labours (Kirkham 1989).

Green and colleagues (1990) found that information was of great importance to women at every stage of their labour, those who were kept informed of non-emergency decisions during labour were more likely to be satisfied with their birth experience.

Continuous support in labour Hodnett (1994) reviewed eleven studies on 'Support from care givers during childbirth' with the objective of assessing the effects of continuous intrapartum support(social or professional). The results showed that: 'Regardless of whether or not a support person of the woman's own choosing could be present the continuous presence of a trained person who had no prior social bond with the labouring woman reduced the likelihood of medication for pain relief, operative vaginal delivery, and a 5-minute Apgar score of less than seven'. Furthermore, 'In a setting that did not permit the presence of significant others, the presence of a trained support person also reduced the likelihood of Caesarean delivery' (Hodnett 1994).

These findings are of particular significance to midwives who, as 'trained supporters' can re-evaluate the way in which they care for and support women during labour. From the available evidence it would appear that women have better physical and emotional labour outcomes if they have continuous support from caregivers, if they are involved in the decision making about their labour and are informed about the progress of their labour. Midwives are in a unique position to make a significant difference to the outcome of a woman's labour. To make that difference midwives must move towards the provision of care which is not fragmented. To provide continuous support would involve a change in the organisation of midwifery care, so that less time is spent on non-midwifery activities and more on the support of women during labour (McNiven & Hodnett 1992). The opportunity for change is made clear in the pages of the report 'Changing childbirth' (Expert Maternity Group 1993). Midwives must seize the challenge of the change if they are to continue to meet the needs of childbearing women and their families.

■ Recommendations for clinical practice in the light of currently available evidence

1. Midwives should ensure that the woman has continuous support from a midwife in labour as such support reduces labour interventions. In addition there is a reduction in the need for analgesia and the neonatal outcome is improved.
2. Women should be kept informed of their progress in labour and included in the decision making process. This will help them to be satisfied with the outcome of their labour even when intervention is necessary.
3. Food and fluids should not be withheld from low risk women in normal labour, as research suggests this affects outcome physiologically and psychologically.
4. Those factors which induce stress in women during labour should be minimised, as a woman's long term emotional health may be compromised by the experience.
5. Midwives should ensure that their knowledge and skills are fully up-to-date, and that they are able care for women both in the community and in the hospital environment.

■ Practice check

- How effective are you at discussing with a woman the choices available to her for pregnancy and childbirth?
- Do you practice in such a way that your clients have continuity of care?
- Do you start a birth plan with the woman at her booking interview and is the plan regularly updated as her pregnancy progresses?
- Do the women in your care have continuous support during labour?

- Are the emotional needs of the women you care for in labour identified and met?
- Do you allow low risk women in normal labour to eat and drink if they wish?
- Have you reflected on the care you are offering women? Have you used the results of your reflection to begin to change your practice?
- Have you discussed with your Supervisor of Midwives the support you are likely to need from her in order to change areas of your practice?
- Have you read the report of the Expert Maternity Group (1993) 'Changing childbirth'? What part are you going to take in the implementation of the recommendations of this report?

■ References

Bohus B, de Kloet ER 1979 Behavioural effects of neuropeptides and corticosteroids. In Jones MT (ed) Interaction within the brain-pituitary-adrenocortical system. Academic Press, New York.

Bowes WA Jr 1992 Labour support: many unanswered questions remain. Birth 19 (March): 38–9

Brown S, Lumley J 1994 Satisfaction with care in labour and birth: a survey of 790 Australian women. Birth 21(1): 4–13

Bryar R 1991 Research and individualised care in midwifery. In Robinson S, Thomson AM (eds) Midwives, research and childbirth Vol 2. Chapman & Hall, London

Bryce FC, Clayton JK, Rand RJ, Beck F, Farquharson DIM, Jones SE 1990 General practitioner obstetrics in Bradford. British Medical Journal 300: 725–7

Burnard P 1990 Learning human skills: 98. Heinemann Nursing, Oxford

Campbell R 1990 The place of birth. In Alexander J, Levy V, Roch S (eds) Intrapartum care: a research-based approach. Macmillan, Basingstoke

Campbell R, Macfarlane A 1987 Where to be born? The debate and the evidence. National Perinatal Epidemiology Unit, Oxford

Campbell R, Macfarlane A 1990 Recent debate on the place of birth. In Garcia J, Kilpatrick R, Richards M. (eds) The politics of maternity care. Clarendon Press, Oxford

Campbell R, Macfarlane A, Cavenagh S 1991 Choice and chance in low risk maternity care. British Medical Journal 303: 1487–8

Crawford JS 1978 Principles and practice of obstetric anaesthesia 4th edn. Blackwell Scientific Publications, Oxford

Crawford JS 1986 Maternal mortality from Mendelson's syndrome. Lancet 1: 920–21

Currell R 1990 The organisation of midwifery care. In Alexander J, Levy V, Roch S (eds) Antenatal Care: a research-based approach. (Midwifery Practice Vol 2). Macmillan, Basingstoke

Department of Health 1994 Report on confidential enquiries into maternal deaths in the United Kingdom 1988–1990. HMSO, London

Department of Health and Social Security 1970 Domiciliary midwifery and maternity bed needs (Peel report). HMSO, London

Dimond B 1993 Client autonomy and choice. Modern Midwife 3(1): 15–16

Drayton S 1990 Midwifery care in the first stage of labour. In Alexander J, Levy V, Roch S (eds) Intrapartum care: a research-based approach (Midwifery Practice Vol 2). Macmillan, Basingstoke

Expert Maternity Group 1993 Changing childbirth. HMSO, London

Flanagan A 1992 Giving birth on an egg. London Times, December 17

Fleissig A 1993 Are women given enough information by staff during labour and delivery? Midwifery 9: 70–75

Flint C 1984 Cosiness in the delivery suite. Nursing Times 80(24): 28–30

Flint C 1991 The Know Your Midwife scheme. In Robinson S, Thomson AM (eds) Midwives, research and childbirth Vol 2. Chapman & Hall, London

Flint C, Poulengeris P 1987 The 'Know your midwife' report. Privately printed; available from 49 Peckarmans Wood, Sydenham Hill, London SE26 6RZ

Garcia J, Garforth S, Ayers S 1986 Midwives confined? Labour ward policies and routines. Research and the Midwife Conference Proceedings: 74–80

Garforth S, Garcia J 1989 Hospital admission practices. In Chalmers I, Enkin M, Keirse MJNC (eds) Effective care in pregnancy and childbirth: Oxford University Press, Oxford

Grant J 1990 Nutrition and hydration in labour. In Alexander J, Levy V, Roch S (eds) Intrapartum care: a research-based approach (Midwifery Practice Vol 2). Macmillan, Basingstoke

Green JM, Coupland VA, Kitzinger JV 1990 Expectations,experiences and psychological outcomes of childbirth: a prospective study of 825 women. Birth 17: 15–24

Hall J 1993 Power games in midwifery. Midwives Chronicle 106(1269): 375

Hauxwell B, Tanner S 1994 Developing an integrated midwifery service. British Journal of Midwifery 2(1): 33–6

Hinchliff S, Montague S 1989 Physiology for nursing practice. Baillière Tindall, London

Hodnett ED 1994 Support from caregivers during childbirth. In Enkin MW, Keirse MJNC, Renfrew MJ, Neilson JP (eds) Pregnancy and childbirth module: Cochrane database of systematic reviews: review no. 03871. Cochrane Updates on Disk, Disk Issue 1, Oxford

House of Commons Health Committee 1992 Second report: Maternity Services Vol 1. HMSO, London

James J 1990 Being a birth attendant. New Generation 9(2): 22–5

Johnson C, Keirse MJNC, Enkin M, Chalmers I 1989 Nutrition and hydration in labour. In Chalmers I, Enkin MW, Keirse MJNC Effective care in pregnancy and childbirth: 827–32. Oxford University Press, Oxford

Jowitt M 1993 Childbirth unmasked: 47–71. Hartnolls Ltd, Cornwall

Keirse MJNC, Enkin M, Lumley J 1989 Social and professional support during childbirth. In Chalmers I, Enkin MW, Keirse MJNC Effective care in pregnancy and childbirth: 805–14. Oxford University Press, Oxford

Kennell J, Marshall K, McGrath S, Robertson S, Hinkley C 1991 Continuous emotional support during labour in a US hospital. Journal of American Medical Association 265(17): 2197–201

Kings Fund Centre 1993 NHS maternity care: choice, continuity and change – a consensus conference March 4th & 5th 1993. Department of Health, London

Kirkham MJ 1983 Labouring in the dark: limitations on the giving of information to enable patients to orientate themselves to the likely events and timescale of labour. In Wilson-Barnett J (ed) Nursing research: Ten studies in patient care. John Wiley, Chichester

Kirkham MJ 1986 A feminist perspective in midwifery. In Webb C (ed) Feminist practice in women's health care. John Wiley, Chichester

Kirkham MJ 1989 Midwives and information giving during labour. In Robinson S, Thomson AM (eds) Midwives, research and childbirth Vol 1. Chapman & Hall, London

Kirkham MJ 1993 Communication in midwifery. In Alexander J, Levy V, Roch S (eds) Midwifery practice: a research-based approach. Macmillan, Basingstoke

Kitzinger S 1987 Freedom and choice in childbirth. Penguin, Harmondsworth

Klaus MH, Kennell JH, Robertson SS, Sosa R 1986 Effects of social support during parturition on maternal and infant morbidity. British Journal of Medicine 2930: 585–7

Klein M, Elbourne D, Lloyd F 1985 Booking for maternity care, a comparison of two systems. Occasional Paper 31. Royal College of General Practitioners, London

Klein M, Lloyd I, Redman C, Bull M, Turnbull AC 1983 A comparison of low-risk women booked for delivery in two systems of care. Parts 1 and 2. British Journal of Obstetrics and Gynaecology 90: 118–22, 123–8

Lederman RP, Lederman E, Work BA Jr, McCann DS 1978 The relationship of maternal anxiety, plasma catecholamines, and plasma cortisol to progress in labour. American Journal of Obstetrics and Gynecology 78: 495

Lederman RP, Lederman E, Work BA Jr, McCann DS 1985 Anxiety and epinephrine in multiparous women in labour: relationship to duration of labour and fetal heart rate pattern. American Journal of Obstetrics and Gynecology 153: 870–77.

Lewis C 1986 Becoming a father. Open University Press, Milton Keynes.

Ludka L 1987 Fasting during labor. Paper presented at the International Confederation of Midwives 21st Congress in the Hague, August 1987

Mander R 1993 Who chooses the choices? Modern Midwife 3: 23–5.

Maternity Services Advisory Committee 1982 Maternity care in action, Part 1: Antenatal Care: a guide to good practice and a plan for action. HMSO, London

McNiven P, Hodnett E 1992 Supporting women in labour: a work sampling study of the activities of labour and delivery nurses. Birth 19(1): 3–8

Mehl LE 1978 The outcome of home delivery: research in the United States. In Kitzinger S, Davis JA (eds) The place of birth, Oxford University Press, Oxford

Mendelson CL 1946 The aspiration of stomach contents into the lungs during obstetric anesthesia. American Journal of Obstetrics and Gynecology 52: 191–205

Methven R 1990 Recording an obstetric history or relating to a pregnant woman? A study of the antenatal booking interview. In Robinson S, Thomson AM (eds) Midwives, research and childbirth Vol 1. Chapman & Hall, London

Niven CA 1985 How helpful is the presence of the husband at childbirth? Journal of Reproduction and Infant Psychology 3: 45–53

Odent M 1984 Birth reborn. Souvenir Press, London

Page L 1993 Redefining the midwife's role: changes needed in practice. British Journal of Midwifery 1(1): 21–4

Pickrell MD, Marshall T 1989 A retrospective cohort study of women presenting with a birth plan. Abstracts: RCOG Silver Jubilee British Congress of Obstetrics and Gynaecology. Royal College of Obstetricians and Gynaecologists, London

Prentice A, Walton SM 1989 Outcome of pregnancies referred to a general practitioner maternity unit in a district hospital. British Medical Journal 299: 1090–92

Read M, Garcia J 1989 Women's views of care during pregnancy and childbirth. In Enkin MW, Keirse MJNC, Chalmers I (eds) Effective care in pregnancy and childbirth: 131–42. Oxford University Press, Oxford

Roberts RB, Shirley MA 1976 The obstetrician's role in reducing the risk of aspiration pneumonitis. With particular reference to the use of oral antacids. American Journal of Obstetrics and Gynecology 124: 611–17

Robinson S 1989 Caring for childbearing women: the interrelationship between midwifery and medical responsibilities.

In Robinson S, Thomson AM (eds) Midwives, research and childbirth Vol 1. Chapman & Hall, London

Robinson S, Golden J, Bradley S 1983 A study of the role and responsibilities of the midwife. Nursing Education Research Unit, Report No 1. Chelsea College, University of London

Romney ML 1980 Predelivery shaving: an unjustified assault? Journal of Obstetrics and Gynaecology 1: 33–5

Romney ML, Gordon H 1981 Is your enema really necessary? British Medical Journal 282: 1269–71

Sangala V, Dunster G, Bohin S, Osbourne JP 1990 Perinatal mortality rates in isolated general practitioner maternity units. British Medical Journal 30: 418–20

Shearer ML 1985 Five year prospective study of risk of booking for home birth. British Medical Journal 201: 1478–80

Simkin P 1986 Stress, pain and catecholamines in labour. Parts 1 & 2: Stress associated with childbirth events: a pilot survey of new mothers. Birth 13: 234–40

Simkin P 1991 Just another day in a woman's life? Part 1: Women's long-term perceptions of their first birth experience. Birth 18(4): 203–10

Simkin P 1992 Just another day in a woman's life? Part II: Nature and consistency of women's long-term memories of their first birth experiences. Birth 19(2): 64–81

Smoleniec JS, James DK 1992 Does having a birth plan affect operative delivery rate? Journal of Obstetrics and Gynaecology 12(6): 394–7

Social Services Committee 1980 Perinatal and neonatal mortality: Second Report, June 19. HMSO, London

Sosa R, Kennell JH, Klaus M, Robertson S, Urrutia J 1980 The effect of a supportive companion on perinatal problems, length of labor and mother-infant interaction. New England Journal of Medicine 303: 597–600

Summersgill P 1993 Couvade – the retaliation of marginalised fathers. In Alexander J, Levy V, Roch S (eds) Midwifery practice: a research-based approach. Macmillan, Basingstoke

Swift L 1991 Labour and fasting. Nursing Times 87(48): 64–5

Swinnerton T 1990 The best laid plans . . . Nursing Times 86(23): 70–71

Taylor A 1986 Maternity services: the consumer's view. Journal of the Royal College of General Practitioners 36: 157–60

Taylor M 1991 Providing emotional support. Nursing Times 87(22): 66

Tew M 1987 Is home birth less safe? Paper presented at the First International Conference on Home Birth, October 24th and 25th, Wembley Conference Centre, London

Webb C 1986 Feminist practice in women's health care. John Wiley, Chichester

Woolet A, Dosanjh-Matwala N 1990 Asian women's experiences of childbirth in East London: the support of fathers and female relatives. Journal of Reproduction and Infant Psychology 1: 37–46

Wolf F 1990 Great expectations (birth plans and how they can place a strain on a labouring woman). Parents Nov: 36–8

Wraight A, Ball J, Seccombe I, Stock J 1993 Mapping team midwifery. Institute of Manpower Studies, Brighton

Zuspan FP, Cibils LA, Pose SV 1962 Myometrial and cardiovascular response to alterations in plasma epinephrine and norepinephrine. American Journal of Obstetrics and Gynecology 84: 841–51

■ Suggested further reading

Brown S, Lumley J 1994 Satisfaction with care in labour and birth: a survey of 790 Australian women. Birth 21(1): 4–13

Grant J 1990 Nutrition and hydration in labour. In Alexander J Levy V, Roch S (eds) Intrapartum care: a research-based approach (Midwifery Practice Vol 2). Macmillan, Basingstoke

Keirse MJNC, Enkin M, Lumley J 1989 Social and professional support during childbirth. In Chalmers I, Enkin MW, Keirse MJNC, (eds) Effective care in pregnancy and childbirth: 805–14. Oxford University Press, Oxford

Ludka L, Roberts C 1993 Eating and drinking in labour: a literature review. Journal of Nurse-Midwifery 38(4): 199–207

Simkin P 1991 Just another day in a woman's life? Part 1, women's long-term perceptions of their first birth experience. Birth 18(4): 203–10

Simkin P 1992 Just another day in a woman's life? Part II: nature and consistency of women's long-term memories of their first birth experiences. Birth 19(2): 64–81

Chapter 3

Disability, pregnancy and parenting

Elaine Carty

Many authors argue that ideologies of motherhood suggest that all women want children (Barnard 1975; Bilton *et al* 1987; Tong 1989). Fine and Asch (1988) note, however, that women with disabilities are expected to forego mothering in the interests of the child. Fears that the disability will be handed on to the child, or that the children might be psychologically harmed, deprived or burdened are often expressed in both the lay and professional communities. Consequently women with disabilities who choose to parent often face negative attitudes from the health professionals they encounter. As midwives we must be aware of our own values and attitudes regarding the rights and responsibilities of childbearing before we can support the pregnant woman who has a disability or chronic illness as she explores the meaning of the pregnancy, works through the challenges of pregnancy, labour and birth, and adapts to her role as mother. Midwives have the potential to strengthen a woman in her ability to give birth and parent in a society that may not be 100 per cent supportive of her decision to do so.

Knowledge about disability and pregnancy, birth and early parenting is increasing as more research is carried out and clinical experience is gained. The purpose of this chapter is to present an overview of our knowledge with respect to childbearing with a disability, and the implications for midwifery practice. Space limitations prevent a thorough examination of all disabilities and chronic illnesses so this chapter will focus on the following disabling conditions: rheumatoid arthritis, spinal cord injury, vision and hearing impairment and multiple sclerosis. Recommendations for clinical practice that are specific to each condition will be listed under the heading for that condition; general recommendations will appear at the end of the chapter.

■ It is assumed that you are already aware of the following:

- The pathophysiology and effects of rheumatoid arthritis, spinal cord injury, vision and hearing impairment and multiple sclerosis;
- That women with disabilities and their families have a sophisticated working knowledge of their disability, its effects and its management (Thorne 1990; 1993).

■ Rheumatoid arthritis

Rheumatoid arthritis (RA) is a systemic inflammatory disorder which causes pain and swelling of the joints, particularly the smaller peripheral joints of the hands and wrists. RA occurs in all races worldwide, affecting women three times as often as men. The prevalence of RA (0.5–2.0 per cent, depending on the criteria used) increases with age, but its onset is generally during the childbearing years (Trock & Craft 1992).

Over the past 50 years, studies of the relationship of arthritis and pregnancy have demonstrated that pregnancy results in a remission of symptoms for approximately 75 per cent of women (Persellin 1977; Ostensen & Husby 1983; Spector & Da Silva 1992). Because the improvement of symptoms is independent of the type of joint involvement, disease duration, number of children, or sex of the fetus, it is hard to predict which women will experience a remission (Ostensen & Husby 1983). Therefore, pregnancy itself is usually not a problem for women with RA; the difficult time is the first year postpartum. Up to 90 per cent of women can expect their symptoms to flare up in the early postpartum period (Ostensen & Rugelsjoen 1992); the flare may last from a few weeks to several months.

Because drug therapy is an essential part of the treatment plan for women with arthritis, the approach to drug use presents a challenge for the 25 per cent of women who will not experience an antepartum remission and for the 90 per cent of women whose flare up may occur during the time in which they are breastfeeding. The salicylates are the drugs which are used most frequently to reduce symptoms. The most frequent dosage in pregnancy is 650 mg, twice or three times daily. It is usually withdrawn four weeks before term because of the risk to the newborn of haemorrhage due to decreased platelet count. Because salicylates accumulate in breast milk, they should not be used by lactating women (Trock & Craft 1992). Women with RA may also be taking nonsteroidal anti-inflammatory drugs which should also be stopped four weeks prior to delivery (Ostensen & Husby 1988). Potential side-effects include prolonged gestation and labour, decreased uteroplacental circulation and premature closure of the ductus arteriosus (Buckley & Kulb 1993). Intramuscular gold therapy has been used safely during pregnancy and lactation (Ostensen & Husby 1983), however, there is one case report of congenital malformation after gold use (Rogers *et al* 1980). Those women on corticosteroid therapy should be maintained during pregnancy and lactation on the lowest possible dose (< 30 mg/day) (Snyder & Snyder 1978).

The needs of the new mother who has a flare up of rheumatoid arthritis can be many. She must cope with pain and fatigue which affect all aspects of her daily life. Ostensen and Rugelsjoen (1992), in a study of 57 women with rheumatic disease, identified aspects of child care which were most difficult. Moving or removing the child from the cot, playpen and car seat was difficult for 70 per cent of the women who had rheumatoid arthritis; bathing and dressing was identified as difficult by 60 per cent. It is during this time that women may wonder about their decision to become a parent and express guilt feelings about not being able to do what 'other' mothers do (Carty & Conine 1988). Many women have said that they felt unprepared for what to expect and had to rely on family and friends for information and support (Conine *et al* 1986, 1987; Ostensen & Rugelsjoen 1992). Even though the studies to date have been done with small samples and with women with varying degrees of disability, the results have identified consistent themes: the need for information and support.

□ **Rheumatoid arthritis: recommendations for clinical practice**

1. Information about the effect of rheumatoid arthritis and drug therapy on the pregnancy, birth, postpartum period, and the newborn, and the effect of pregnancy on the course of RA should be offered to women prior to pregnancy, or in the early pregnancy period.
2. Ways in which the woman can pace herself, so that she can have both systemic and joint rest, should be discussed with her. In order to reduce fatigue, it is recommended (Rodnan & Schumacker 1983) that the woman:
   • wears braces to support her joints;

- has two rest periods per day;
- sleeps 8–10 hours per night if possible;
- sits whenever possible during the day.
3. In discussion with the woman the midwife should also focus on how rest must be balanced with exercise to reduce stiffness, prevent muscle atrophy and the loss of joint mobility. Encourage the woman to have a regular exercise routine that she follows daily. Swimming is an excellent exercise for women with RA as long they avoid chilling and becoming overtired.
4. Offer suggestions to make dressing (for both herself and her baby) less difficult. Maternity and baby clothes may have to be altered with Velcro® openings or large ring zippers. Antique buttonhooks are helpful to manipulate small buttons. Front closure bras may need to be adapted with Velcro®.
5. Assist the couple with suggestions to make sexual activity as pleasurable as possible. Planning the time of sexual activity (even if it means getting a babysitter) will allow preparation that might be required: using an analgesic to reduce discomfort; taking a warm bath or shower to reduce joint stiffness; or incorporating 'range of motion' exercises and light massage into sexual pleasuring (Klinger 1980).
6. Discuss with the family the importance of assistance with baby care and household care. Because of postpartum pain and fatigue, this is a time when many women feel they have made a wrong decision in having a baby. A thorough discussion with family members of what to expect, and of all the supports that will need to be in place, will assist the woman in focusing on her abilities, not her disabilities.
7. Assist the mother to find a network or support group of other mothers with rheumatic disease.

■ Spinal cord injury

What little we know about spinal cord injury and pregnancy has come from two sources. The first of these is the scientific literature, which has focused primarily on outcomes (Wanner *et al* 1987; Baker *et al* 1992; Charlifue *et al* 1992; Cross *et al* 1992). The second source is the lay and social science literature which has described the experiences women have had during the pregnancy and postpartum periods (Morris 1989; Campion 1990; Rogers & Matsumura 1991; Haseltine *et al* 1993).

Based on the evidence from published reports, women with spinal cord injury have good outcomes and should not be discouraged from becoming pregnant for health and safety reasons. Nonetheless, certain complications arise frequently in the antepartum period. Urinary tract infection has been reported to be as high as 100 per cent in women with indwelling catheters and 50 per cent in women who are catheterised intermittently (Cross *et al* 1992) In Baker and colleagues' 1992 study, 10 of 11 women experienced urinary tract infection. Three of the women experienced the more severe complication of pyelonephritis.

There is a serious potential for skin breakdown in women with spinal cord injury. Oedema, increased weight, altered centre of gravity and difficulties in transferring can all result in the development of pressure points. This problem has been noted in all research reports.

Many women are on medication to control spasticity and spasms. It is suggested that a thorough assessment of the woman's situation be carried out so that the dosage of these medications be reduced before pregnancy is undertaken if possible (Kuemmerle & Bredel 1984; Niebyl 1988). Diazepam (Valium), which is commonly used to control spasms, has been known to result in withdrawal symptoms in the baby (Cross *et al* 1992). There is also a reported increase in the incidence of cleft palate in babies of mothers on Diazepam (Safra & Oakley 1975; Saxen 1975).

Preterm labour has been reported to be more frequent in women with spinal cord injury (Verduyn 1986; Charlifue *et al* 1992). Yet this has not been the case in our experience in Vancouver (Effer 1994) or in the study by Baker *et al* (1992). More data are required to determine the incidence of preterm labour in spinal cord injured women as the current approach to care, which often involves long periods of hospitalisation or home care with uterine monitoring, may not be appropriate.

Autonomic hyperreflexia (AH) occurs in up to 85 per cent of women with lesions at or above the sixth thoracic vertebra (Baker *et al* 1992; Charlifue *et al* 1992; Cross *et al* 1992). AH is an exaggerated response of the sympathetic nervous system, characterised by an elevated blood pressure, profuse sweating and flushed face, apprehension, and nasal stuffiness or obstruction. AH is triggered by somatic and visceral stimulation below the level of the lesion: a full bowel or bladder; a pelvic examination; or uterine contractions in labour. Some practitioners may choose to treat symptoms only, while others may choose to use suppressive therapy with antihypertensives or regional anaesthesia. Baker and colleagues note that the potential for autonomic hyperreflexia is often not recognised by caregivers and the appropriate treatment measures not instituted, thus resulting in unnecessary morbidity and mortality.

More recent studies have also noted that the rate of caesarean delivery is no higher than the rate in the general population (Baker *et al* 1992; Charlifue *et al* 1992). Often women with spinal cord injury find that both lay individuals and health care professionals, who have little information about outcomes for women with spinal cord injury, assume that women with spinal cord injuries will need a caesarean section. If a woman is advised during the pregnancy period that she will need a caesarean, she should seek a second opinion to be sure that it is truly indicated (Carty *et al* 1993a).

The postpartum experience of women with spinal cord injury has been poorly documented in the health care literature. Only recently have women begun to write about their experiences and consequently to provide some information for others to use (Morris 1989; Campion 1990; Rogers & Matsumura 1991; Haseltine *et al* 1993). The thrust of all these authors is positive; they identify the potential difficulties with parenting and suggest strategies.

☐ **Spinal cord injury: recommendations for clinical practice**

1. Women with spinal cord injury have been through a strenuous period of rehabilitation during which they have learned to care for themselves and very clearly identify their needs. They have adapted their living evironment to become as independent as possible. Caregivers must always respect the woman as the primary source of information about how to proceed.

2. Women with spinal cord injury are used to monitoring their own health with respect to urinary tract infection, but may need the information that their susceptibility to infection will be even higher during pregnancy due to the effect of progesterone on the ureters. Encourage fluid intake including acidic fluids such as cranberry, prune and other fresh fruit juices. Suggest bladder emptying before and after sexual intercourse. Encourage women to discuss with their doctor the possibility of a prophylactic antimicrobial medication regime.

3. To prevent skin breakdown, it is important for the woman to implement strategies such as frequent changes

of position, regular inspection of the skin, and careful attention to the padding and size of the wheelchair. During the postpartum period, lochial flow and sanitary pads can be irritating to the skin. Frequent perineal care is essential in the early postpartum days. Commercial diapers may be more comfortable than perineal pads. If there is an episiotomy, the site should be examined regularly for breakdown. Bath or shower temperatures should be carefully checked in order to prevent burns.

4. Assist the woman to maintain her bowel regime, recognising that this may be difficult particularly in late pregnancy when constipation is common for many women. Maintenance of haemoglobin levels through food intake rather than iron supplementation will be helpful. Advice about foods which are high in iron, and on increasing fluid intake as well as fibre and bulk, will assist in the prevention of constipation.

5. Most women are able to identify the kinds of activities which can stimulate autonomic hyperreflexia; midwives should be particularly careful with the pelvic examination and should help the woman to avoid impacted bowels. Labour often precipitates hyperreflexia, and since it more often occurs when the woman is in the supine position, a semi-sitting position should be used if possible. Epidural anaesthesia is often used as a preventative measure as labour progresses.

■ Sensory impairment

Very little research is available on the particular needs and experiences of women with low vision or hearing impairment. Because these disabilities do not affect pregnancy outcome *per se*, medical journals are devoid of information. However, because of the difficulties which arise when communication is hampered by a vision or hearing impairment, midwives and nurses have written of their experiences so that care can be more sensitive (Cranston, undated; Campion 1990; Kelsall *et al* 1992).

□ Visual impairment

A woman with a visual impairment, like all women with a disability, may be fearful of how her decision to become a parent will be received by family and health professionals. This concern often comes from her awareness that in our society, terms such as 'blind drunk', 'blind faith' and 'the blind leading the blind' suggest that blindness is associated with ignorance and incompetence (Carty *et al* 1990).

The suggestions for clinical practice come from the author's experience of working with women who are blind and from the few anecdotal articles available.

☐ **Visual impairment: recommendations for clinical practice**

1. The midwife may want to spend more time on a one-to-one basis with her client as detailed descriptions of many aspects of the childbirth process may be necessary. Tactile models, such as the doll and pelvis, a knitted uterus (NCT or ICEA Teaching Aid, see Resources), and the raised cervical dilatation chart will help in explaining the process of labour and delivery (Carty *et al* 1993b).
2. Assisting the woman to palpate her abdomen and identify fetal parts, listening to the fetal heart for a longer period of time and focusing on fetal movements will help the woman who is blind to get to know her baby prenatally (Carty *et al* 1993b).
3. A tour of the hospital or birth centre is important for the woman to orient herself by identifying boundaries to the space and potential obstacles. Special arrangements may need to be made if the woman requests the presence of her guide dog.
4. Because there are a number of different workers in any health care agency, it is important to remember that everyone needs to introduce her or himself to the woman by name and by function. Information on name tags is not accessible to the blind or partially sighted woman.
5. During the birth it might helpful for the woman to feel her baby's head as it emerges, and to receive the baby onto her abdomen immediately so she can run her hands over the baby. The initial examination of the baby should be done while the woman has the baby with her, with clear descriptive accounts of every aspect so that she can picture the baby in her mind. The midwife can assist the mother in her attachment process by describing the characteristics of her baby, the expressions, the movements and behaviours which the baby exhibits (Carty *et al* 1993b).

☐ **Hearing impairment**

Individuals who experience hearing loss speak of their disability as an 'invisible disability'; it is only after trying to communicate with someone with a hearing loss, that the disability becomes evident. Kelsall and colleagues (1992) clearly outline types of hearing loss and strategies for the midwife to use as she works with women with hearing impairment during pregnancy, birth and postpartum. Some research has been done recently on the parenting skills of deaf parents. These studies have indicated that parents carry out their parenting skills in a most positive way (Jones *et al* 1989). One study, (Rienzi 1988) found that families in which the parents were deaf were very adaptable in their roles and expectations, and that hearing children of deaf parents had a greater percentage of their ideas accepted in the family than did hearing children of hearing parents.

☐ **Hearing impairment: recommendations for clinical practice**

1. The midwife needs to determine the way in which the woman is most comfortable communicating; writing, wearing a hearing aid, lip-reading, finger spelling, sign language, or using an interpreter. If the woman prefers using an interpreter, she should consider using the same person throughout the pregnancy, labour and delivery and the postpartum period.
2. During the pregnancy, the midwife should let the hospital know that her client is hearing impaired and that an interpreter will be accompanying the woman for all procedures and for birth. The records should be clearly marked.
3. Because the majority of women do lip-read, the midwife will want to: obtain the woman's attention before speaking; face the woman; speak slowly but not overmouth words; repeat and rephrase as necessary; remain patient; and avoid analgesics that may cause drowsiness, making it difficult for the woman to concentrate on lip-reading.
4. Provide a tour of the hospital or birth centre and determine which labour room or postpartum room would be most suitable (quiet so as not to interfere with the hearing aid, or close to the midwife's station for reassurance).
5. Watch for facial expressions during procedures and labour as the woman may not be able to communicate her

discomfort or concern. Because she cannot hear the baby's heartbeat she will need reassurance that all is going well. Position her for birth so that she can see the midwife's face clearly. Wear a transparent mask if one must be worn at all.

6. Provide as much literature as possible for all aspects of pregnancy care and baby care. Provide information on baby alarm devices for the hearing impaired (Conine *et al* 1988).

■ Multiple sclerosis

Multiple sclerosis (MS) is a chronic neurological disease characterised by progressive demyelination of the central nervous system (Miller & Hens 1993). The exact cause of MS is unknown. Onset of MS symptoms tends to occur between the ages of 20 and 40. Prevalence of MS is 1.8 times higher in women than men. There is no cure so, once a woman is diagnosed, she is faced with the reality of life with a chronic illness. Since many of these woman are also of childbearing age, they must also face the decision of whether or not to have a child.

MS is no longer classified as one illness, but is now understood to come in mild, moderate, severe forms, and to follow either a cyclical pattern (remission/exacerbation/remission), or a pattern of slow and steady progression towards severe disability (Cook 1990). Current research done by Weinshenker and colleagues (1989) indicates that pregnancy does not affect the long term course of MS. Today, only women with the most severe form of MS are advised to avoid pregnancy, and this type of MS happens less frequently in women than it does in men (Weinshenker *et al* 1989).

Women with MS will have different needs according to the severity of their disease. For example, a woman with mild MS will have less specialised needs than a woman with moderate or severe MS who has extensive nervous damage. Women with moderate to severe MS can have any combination of symptoms ranging from blurred vision, muscle weakness, spasms, or ataxia leading to the use of a cane or wheelchair, poor bladder control (urgency and/or incontinence), alteration in bowel function (constipation or incontinence), or sexual dysfunction (lack of vaginal lubrication, genital insensitivity, hypersensitivity to touch, clitoral engorgement) (Fox *et al* 1990). Each woman will adapt to pregnancy, delivery, and childbearing in her own unique way and the kind of care she needs will depend on the symptoms she experiences.

Research indicates that most women with MS who experience an exacerbation in association with pregnancy do so in the first 3–6 months after the birth and may be temporarily unable to care for their infant (Birk *et al* 1988; Nelson *et al* 1988). Bernardi and colleagues (1991) found, however, that the exacerbation rate during the postpartum period was still less than the rate during non-pregnancy related times. Pregnancy therefore, seems to have a protective effect (Bernardi *et al* 1991). Nelson and colleagues (1988) also studied the relationship between multiple sclerosis exacerbation and breastfeeding and concluded that there was no effect. Breastfeeding does require getting up several times during the night, and muscle strength and co-ordination. Rogers and Matsumura (1991) interviewed several women with MS who reported that breastfeeding worsened their fatigue. Therefore, when discussing infant feeding prior to delivery, a woman should be encouraged to weigh carefully her desire to breastfeed with her need for rest in the postpartum period.

A recent study of the interaction patterns of mothers with multiple sclerosis and their daughters aged 8–12 years (Crist 1993), identified no differences when compared with mothers without MS and their daughters with respect to receptiveness, directiveness and dissuasiveness in both play and work related tasks. These findings contradict earlier literature which suggests negative child-parent interactions in parents with a chronic illness (Buck & Hohmann 1983), and perhaps reflects changing attitudes and support services available to women today.

While many women with disabilities will not choose to have genetic counselling, the midwife should explore the advantages and disadvantages of this technology with any woman with MS who is considering another pregnancy. Current research shows that there is a tendency for MS to run in families. Parents with MS should be aware that their offspring face a lifetime 3–5 per cent chance of developing MS compared to the 0.1 per cent chance that faces the general population (Sadovnick 1984).

□ **Multiple sclerosis: recommendations for clinical practice**

1. Co-ordination of care may be an especially important task for the midwife caring for a woman with MS. Such a woman will usually be involved with several health professionals, for example she may see a neurologist, nutritionist and, if her MS is moderate to severe, a neurological

physiotherapist for exercises to help minimise the weakness, spasticity, and ataxia she experiences. She may also see an occupational therapist to help her make adaptations for daily living in her home. Each of these aspects of care is important to the overall management of MS before, during, and after pregnancy.

2. Since fatigue is known to bring exacerbations in MS, the midwife should stress the importance of adequate rest as the cornerstone of care. Strenuous exercise should be avoided. Encourage the woman, instead, to do gentle toning exercises that strengthen the abdomen and pelvic floor. Also to reduce stress and fatigue, it may be helpful for the partner to room-in with the mother postpartum to assist with baby care (British Columbia Women's Hospital and Health Centre Society 1994).

■ General recommendations for clinical practice in the light of currently available evidence

1. *Provide services in settings which are architecturally or physically accessible*

   The midwife should ask the following questions about the surroundings which will be used by her client. Is it possible to approach the building by wheelchair? Is the area outside the entry large enough to allow van parking as many women who use a wheelchair travel by van? Are doors wide enough to allow wheelchair entry? Are door handles of the lever type and at a height which can be reached from a wheelchair? Is the place where childbirth education classes are held accessible? Is it possible for exercise mats to be placed on a raised platform? Can the examining table be lowered for easier transfer? Are labour and postpartum rooms large enough to allow safe transfer from wheelchair to toilet? Are hospital beds fixed with electric controls? Are cots for the newborn adjustable in height? Showers without lips or sills provide the easiest access to water, used for both comfort during labour and regular hygiene. Some birth pools and bathtubs can be made accessible with the use of transfer boards, or stools.

2. *Provide services which are psychologically accessible*

   Physical accessibility by itself is insufficient for the experience of childbirth to be a positive one. The midwife and other members of the health care team should put procedures in place that allow the woman with a disability to know that her needs and concerns will be respected. Every client, when first seeking out services, should be asked if she has a disability or chronic illness which needs special consideration (Task Force 1978). For example, a woman with limited mobility could benefit from some or all of her prenatal visits taking place in her own home; if she needs to go to a clinic or hospital her visit will be easier if she can be met at the door by a porter or volunteer and assisted to the appropriate location. Appointments can be scheduled at a time when the clinic is least busy as it often takes extra time for a woman to remove a brace, do a self-catheterisation or transfer from a wheelchair.

Another aspect of psychological accessibility is the provision of care using a respectful, sensitive communication style. It is important to learn about the disability from the woman, and learn about her specific coping strategies. This involves communicating directly with the woman herself, not asking questions of those accompanying her unless she specifically requests that you do so. She should be asked what assistance she needs before providing help and her permission should be asked before touching her wheelchair or prosthesis (Asrael & Kesselman 1982).

It is important to offer information about sexuality, pregnancy, birth and their impact on the disabling condition without being asked. Information which encourages the woman to choose from options allows her to increase her control. Assisting the woman to build confidence is important. This can be accomplished through careful planning of all aspects of pregnancy and birth and by involving all care providers in a team approach. Some women relate that the health professionals they encounter talk only about the difficulties they foresee and leave the women with the feeling that they doubt their ability to manage pregnancy, birth and parenting (Rogers & Matsumura 1991).

3. *Provide preconception care if possible to assist the woman and her family prior to her decision to become pregnant*
The following areas should be addressed:
- The effects of the condition or disability on pregnancy, labour and birth, and the postpartum period;
- The effects of pregnancy, labour and birth, and the

postpartum period on the condition or disability;
- The effect of specific medications on fetal development;
- Modifications of lifestyle that could enhance health prior to and during the childbearing period;
- Family adjustments that might be necessary because of the pregnancy/disability interrelationship;
- Family planning options to facilitate appropriate timing of pregnancy;
- Resources in the health care and social services systems and optimal timing for their use.

4. *Provide pregnancy care which is sensitive, based on a thorough assessment of physical and psychosocial needs, and well planned*
If the midwife has not had a chance to meet the woman prior to her becoming pregnant, all of the topics noted above will need to be addressed early in pregnancy. Extra time spent documenting a thorough history, assessing the client's needs and resources with respect to employment, housing, finances, and family relationships, and developing a plan for pregnancy and birth and the early postpartum period, can help to eliminate surprises. Relevant information can be shared with other members of the health care team so that each can contribute to the plan for care to avoid gaps and overlap. If a woman is planning a home birth, then less energy needs to go into making the environment accessible for her. If she is planning a hospital birth, however, it can take several weeks of planning to obtain the correct mattress for a woman with spinal cord injury or a toilet adapter for a woman with hip pain. Advanced care planning conferences with various members of hospital staff who will be involved with the care of the midwife's client will be most useful. In the author's experience, continuity of care has been best facilitated by, firstly, admission of the woman to a room on the maternity ward which has been adapted to accommodate wheelchairs in the bathroom and shower and which has room for an extra bed for an experienced caregiver; and, secondly, provision of nursing care by a designated team of nurses whose duty rotations have been adapted so they will provide care on a 24-hour basis during the woman's hospital stay.

Physical examination may be difficult for the woman with a disability or chronic illness. The midwife should do as much of the examination as possible with the woman in the position which is most comfortable for her, or in her

wheelchair if she wishes. She should be asked to bring a
companion with her to the appointment, one who is
familiar with her transfer techniques. If the midwife is
assisting the woman with transfers, time must be taken to
learn the ways which are most comfortable for the woman.
Braces, crutches and wheelchairs should be left close by.

Like most women, she may feel vulnerable during a
breast or pelvic examination. Determine in advance what
kind of draping, if any, she would prefer. The lithotomy
position for pelvic examination is apt to be the most
difficult for a woman with limited mobility to assume. After
determining the extent of a woman's abilities with respect
to positioning, consider doing the pelvic examination in
any of the following positions: knee-chest, diamond shaped
(on back with legs in diamond shape, no stirrups), side-lying,
or modifications of the these positions (Ferreyra & Hughes
1991). If a spasm should occur during the pelvic
examination, the midwife should support the limb or area
in spasm and wait until the spasm has gone away before
proceeding. Spasms can be exaggerated if the woman is
feeling anxious. A close presence, and thorough
explanations can decrease feelings of uncertainty.

5. *Plan for the special needs of labour and birth*
   If the woman is planning a home birth, it is helpful to
   talk through a mock labour with a number of potential
   scenarios so that the midwife and family together
   can determine what personnel and equipment might be
   necessary. It is important to determine what back-up
   supports are available and to communicate with the
   hospital in advance, in case transfer to hospital is
   necessary. It would be useful to review the client's needs
   with the hospital so that the midwife can be reassured that
   her client will be going into an environment with some
   degree of physical and psychological accessibility.

   If the client is planning a hospital birth, the most
   accessible labour room should be identified. A prenatal
   visit to the unit will help a woman with a disability or
   chronic illness to determine whether she is able to
   function in the surroundings and, if not, what adaptations
   would be helpful.

   It may be beneficial if the woman can find another
   woman with a similar disability or who is familiar with the
   disability to act as a labour coach. If that resource is not
   available it may be possible to identify a childbirth

educator, physiotherapist, midwife or nurse who has worked with someone with a particular disability who would be willing to be a supportive companion in labour.

6. *Assist the mother to organise for the many needs of the postpartum period*
Careful planning in the antenatal period will go a long way to help the first few postpartum weeks go as smoothly as possible. Postpartum fatigue is troublesome for all women at this time, but the woman with a disability or chronic illness will be especially hampered by overwhelming feelings of tiredness. Being sure that there is assistance in place in the home is critical if the woman is to feel confident in her ability to parent. During these early weeks the midwife will focus on:
- The postpartum physical condition of the mother;
- Emotional adjustment to parenthood;
- The aids and adaptations required to carry out baby care;
- How to work out a positive relationship with a child care helper;
- Family planning counselling.

(Carty *et al* 1989; Carty *et al* 1993a, 1993b).

□ **Conclusion**

The development of resources for women with disabilities, and an interest on the part of midwives to provide care for this group of women, should result in well informed mothers, whose skills are enhanced to their maximum potential through aids, adaptations and support. Women with disabilities will need to be actively involved in the development of specialised services and in the evaluation of those services; a true midwife-client partnership.

■ **Practice check**

- Consider your own attitudes and beliefs about women with disabilities becoming pregnant. Do you feel it is a woman's right to have children if she wishes, or do you feel there should be certain limitations? Why do you feel the way you do?
- Consider the health care agency where you work. Is it architecturally and psychologically accessible?

● Do you know the resources available in your community which could provide you or your clients with assistance with finances, childcare or adaptive devices for women with disabilities?

☐ **Acknowledgements**

I would like to thank my colleague, Dr Tali Conine, UBC School of Rehabilitation Sciences, for her input into this chapter; and research assistants Angela Holbrook and Lenore Riddell who continually update the database of resources available in the area of disability and childbearing.

■ **References**

Asrael W, Kesselman S 1982 Classes for the disabled. Childbirth Educator 1: 18–23
Baker E, Cardenas D, Benedetti T 1992 Risks associated with pregnancy in spinal cord-injured women. Obstetrics and Gynecology 80(3): 425–8
Barnard J 1975 The future of motherhood. Penguin Books, New York
Bernardi S, Grasso MG, Bertollini R, Onzi F, Fieschi C 1991 The influence of pregnancy on relapses in multiple sclerosis: a cohort study. Acta Neurologica Scandinavia 84: 403–6
Bilton T, Bonnett K, Jones P 1987 Introductory sociology. Macmillan, London
Birk K, Smeltzer S, Rudick R 1988 Pregnancy and multiple sclerosis. Seminars in Neurology 8(3): 205–13.
Bohlin AB, Larsson G 1986 Early identification of infants at risk for institutional care. Journal of Advanced Nursing 11(5): 493–7.
British Columbia Women's Hospital and Health Centre Society 1994 Guidelines for practice. Vancouver, Canada
Buck FM, Hohmann GW 1983 Parental disability and children's adjustment. In Pan EL, Backer TE, Vash CJ (eds) Annual review of rehabilitation vol 3: 203–41. Springer, New York
Buckley K, Kulb NW (eds) 1993 High risk maternity nursing manual 2nd edn: 69–73. Williams & Wilkins, Baltimore
Campion MJ 1990 The baby challenge: a handbook on pregnancy for women with a physical disability. Tavistock/Routledge, London
Carty E, Conine TA, Wood-Johnson F 1986 Rheumatoid arthritis and pregnancy: helping women to meet their needs. Midwives Chronicle 99 (1186): 254–7.
Carty E, Conine TA 1988 Disability and pregnancy: a double dose of disequilibrium. Rehabilitation Nursing 13(2): 85–7
Carty E, Conine TA, Hall L 1990 Comprehensive health promotion for

the pregnant woman who is disabled. Journal of Nurse-Midwifery   35(3): 133–42

Carty E, Conine T, Holbrook A, Riddell L 1993a Guidelines for serving disabled women. Midwifery Today   27 (Autumn): 29–37

Carty E, Conine T, Holbrook A, Riddell L 1993b Childbearing and parenting with a disability or chronic illness. Midwifery Today   28 (Winter): 17–19, 40–42

Charlifue SW, Gerhart JA, Menter RR, Whiteneck GG, Manley MS 1992 Sexual issues of women with spinal cord injuries. Paraplegia   30(3): 192–9

Conine TA, Carty EA, Wood-Johnson F 1986 Provision of preventive maternal health care and childbirth education for disabled women. Canadian Journal of Public Health   77: 123–7.

Conine TA, Carty EA, Wood-Johnson F 1987 Nature and source of information received by primiparas with rheumatoid arthritis on preventive maternal and child care. Canadian Journal of Public Health   78: 393–7

Conine TA, Carty EA, Safarik P 1988 Aids and adaptations for parents with physical or sensory disabilities. School of Rehabilitation Medicine, Vancouver, BC

Cook SD 1990 Handbook of multiple sclerosis. Marcel Dekker, New York

Cranston R (undated) Parenting without vision in 1000 easy lessons. BANANAS, Oakland

Crist P 1993 Contingent interaction during work and play tasks for mothers with multiple sclerosis and their daughters. American Journal of Occupational Therapy   47(2): 121–31

Cross LL, Meythaler JM, Tuel SM, Cross AL 1992 Pregnancy, labor, and delivery post spinal cord injury. Paraplegia   30(12): 890–902

Effer S 1994 Perinatologist. Personal Communication, British Columbia Women's Hospital and Health Centre Society, Vancouver

Ferreyra S, Hughes K 1991 Table manners: A guide to the pelvic examination for disabled women and health care providers 3rd edn. Planned Parenthood Alameda, San Francisco

Fine M, Asch A (eds) 1988 Women with disabilities: essays in psychology, culture and politics. Temple University Press, Philadelphia

Fox M, Harms R, Davis D 1990 Selected neurological complications of pregnancy. Mayo Clinic Proceedings   65(12): 1595–618

Hard S 1987 Documenting the sexual abuse of persons with developmental disabilities. The Committee Exchange 8. Committee on the Sexuality of the Developmentally Disabled, Danville CA

Haseltine FP, Cole SS, Gray DB (eds) 1993 Reproductive issues for persons with physical disabilities. Paul H Brookes, Baltimore

Heighway SM, Kidd-Webster S 1988 Supported parenting: Promoting the welfare of children whose parents are mentally retarded. National Resource Institute on Children and Youth with Handicaps Update   1–2.

Jones E, Strom R, Daniels S 1989 Evaluating the success of deaf parents. American Annals of the Deaf   134(5): 312–16

Kaatz JL 1992 Enhancing the parenting skills of developmentally disabled parents: A nursing perspective. Journal of Community Health Nursing 9(4): 209–19

Kelsall J, King D, O'Grady D 1992 Maternity care for the deaf. Royal National Institute for the Deaf, Manchester

Klinger J (ed) 1980 Self help manual for patients with arthritis. The Arthritis Foundation, Atlanta

Kuemmerle HP, Bredel K (eds) 1984 Clinical pharmacology in pregnancy. Thieme Stratton, New York

Miller CM, Hens M 1993 Multiple sclerosis: a literature review. Journal of Neuroscience Nursing 25(3): 174–9

Morris J (ed) 1989 Able lives: women's experience of paralysis. The women's press, London

Niebyl JR 1988 Drug use in pregnancy. Lea and Febiger, Philadelphia

Nelson L, Franklin G, Jones M 1988 Risk of multiple sclerosis exacerbation during pregnancy and breast-feeding. Journal of the American Medical Association 259(23): 3441–3

Ostensen M 1990 Couselling women with rheumatic disease – how many children are desirable? Scandinavian Journal of Rheumatology 19: 1–5

Ostensen M, Husby G 1983 A prospective clinical trial of the effect of pregnancy on rheumatoid arthritis and ankylosing spondylitis. Arthritis and Rheumatism 26(9): 1155–9

Ostensen M, Rugelsjoen A 1992 Problem areas of the rheumatic mother. American Journal of Reproductive Immunology 28: 254–5

Persellin RH 1977 The effect of pregnancy on rheumatoid arthritis. Bulletin of Rheumatic Diseases 27: 922.

Rienzi B 1988 Influence and adaptability in families with deaf parents and hearing children. American Annals of the Deaf 135(5): 402–8

Rodnan GP, Schumacker HR (eds) 1983 Primer on the rheumatic diseases. The Arthritis Foundation, Atlanta

Rogers JG, Anderson RM, Chow CW, Gillam GL, Markman L 1980 Possible teratogenic effects of gold. Australian Paediatric Journal 16: 194

Rogers J, Matsumura M 1991 Mother to be: a guide to pregnancy and birth for women with disabilities. Demos, New York

Rossier AB, Ruffieux M, Ziegler WH 1969 Pregnancy and labour in high traumatic spinal cord lesions. Paraplegia 7: 210–15

Sadovnick AD 1984 Becoming a parent is a major decision when MS is in the family. MS Canada December: 6–7

Safra JM, Oakley GP 1975 Association between cleft lip with or without cleft palate and neonate exposure to diazepam. Lancet ii: 478–80

Saxen I 1975 Epidemiology of cleft lip and palate. British Journal of Preventive and Social Medicine 29: 103–10

Snyder RD, Snyder D 1978 Corticosteroid for asthma during pregnancy. Annals of Allergy 41: 340

Spector TD, Da Silva JAP 1992 Pregnancy and rheumatoid arthritis: an overview. American Journal of Reproductive Immunology. 28: 222–5

Task Force on Concerns of Physically Disabled Women 1978 Within reach: Providing family planning services to physically disabled women. Human Sciences Press, New York

Thorne, S 1990 Mothers with chronic illness: a predicament of social construction. Health Care for Women International 11: 209–21

Thorne S 1993 Negotiating health care: the social context of chronic illness. Sage, London

Tong R 1989 Feminist thought. Westview Press, San Francisco

Trock D, Craft J 1992 Arthritis and pregnancy. In Reese EA *et al.* (eds) Medicine of the fetus and its mother: 1220–36. JB Lippincott, Toronto

Verduyn WH 1986 Spinal cord injured women, pregnancy, and delivery. Paraplegia 24: 231–40

Wanner WB, Rageth CJ, Zach GA 1987 Pregnancy and autonomic hyperreflexia in spinal cord lesions. Paraplegia 25: 482–90.

Weinshenker BG, Hader W, Carriere BA, Baskerville J, Ebers GC 1989 The influence of pregnancy on disability from multiple sclerosis. Neurology 39(11): 1438–40

■ **Suggested further reading and resources**

Campion MJ 1990 Isobel's baby (video). Arrowhead Publications, London
Deals with one woman's emotional and practical adaptation to motherhood. Can be used to share with women and as a starting point for discussion around the many issues associated with multiple sclerosis and pregnancy. For more information, write to Mukti Campion, 1 Chiswick Staithe, London W4 3TP

Childbearing and parenting program for women with disabilities/ chronic illnesses. For more information, please write to Elaine Carty, University of British Columbia School of Nursing, T206–2211 Wesbrook Mall, Vancouver, BC, V6T 2B5. (604) 822–7444; fax 822–7466

Disability, Pregnancy & Parenthood International. A journal and forum for professionals and parents to exchange information and experience. Arrowhead Publications, 1 Chiswick Staithe, London, W4 3TP

MS Society of Great Britain and Northern Ireland. Has your mum or dad got MS? Nattress House, London Offers useful information to help educate children whose parents have MS.

Parks S 1984 HELP: When the parent is handicapped. VORT Corporation, Palo Alto, CA

■ **Useful addresses**

Multiple Sclerosis Society
25 Effie Road
Fulham
London SW6 IEE
0171 796 6267

National Childbirth Trust: Parentability
Alexandra House
Oldham Terrace
Acton
London W3 6NH
0181 992 8637

Chapter 4

Shoulder dystocia

Terri Coates

We are likely to remember all the cases of shoulder dystocia that we are ever involved with. They are amongst the most terrifying experiences that midwifery or obstetrics has to offer.

It is possible that shoulder dystocia is the least well publicised obstetric emergency. It receives scant coverage in many midwifery and obstetric texts and in some cases is ignored completely. Being an infrequently encountered obstetric emergency, it may be difficult to gain clinical experience in its management.

It is the aim of this chapter to enhance midwives' understanding of the mechanisms involved in shoulder dystocia and the manoeuvres which may be used to help to relieve the problem. Readers may find it useful to have a doll and pelvis within easy reach.

■ It is assumed that you are already aware of the following:

- The anatomy of the pelvic bones and soft tissues;
- Pelvic diameters;
- The mechanism of normal labour and delivery;
- Gross fetal anatomy.

■ Definition and diagnosis

In an address to an obstetrical society in 1954 Professor Morris provided the classic description of shoulder dystocia:

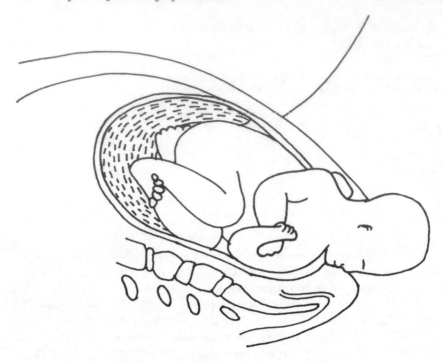

Figure 4.1 Shoulder dystocia: anterior shoulder is stuck at the symphysis pubis, posterior shoulder is wedged into the sacral hollow, the face and chin are burrowing into the perineum

The delivery of the head with or without forceps may have been quite easy, but more commonly there has been a little difficulty in completing the extension of the head. The hairy scalp slides with reluctance. When the forehead has appeared it is necessary to press back the perineum to deliver the face. Fat cheeks eventually emerge. A double chin has to be hooked over the posterior commissure, to which it remains tightly opposed. Restitution seldom occurs spontaneously for the head seems incapable of movement as a result of friction with the girdle of contact at the vulva. . . .

. . . time passes. The child's face becomes suffused. It endeavours unsuccessfully to breathe. Abdominal efforts by the mother or by her attendants produce no advance, gentle head traction is equally unavailing. . . .

. . . Usually equanimity forsakes the attendants. They push, they pull. Alarm increases. Eventually, by greater strength of muscle or some infernal juggle, the difficulty seems to be overcome. . . . It dawns upon the attendants that their anxiety was not ill founded.

Morris 1955: 305

Shoulder dystocia is caused by the failure of the shoulders to spontaneously traverse the pelvis after the delivery of the fetal head (Smeltzer 1986), and results in deliveries which require manoeuvres to deliver the shoulders other than downward traction (Resnik 1980). The cardinal sign that shoulder dystocia has occurred is when the newly delivered head tries to return from whence it came. This is caused by a reverse traction. The posterior shoulder may not have negotiated the pelvic inlet or could be wedged into the hollow of the sacrum, and the anterior shoulder is hooked onto the symphysis pubis. The infant's neck is stretched from the pelvic inlet to the outlet (Smeltzer 1986).

Application of traction to the head at this time serves to impede rather than promote delivery, causing further impaction of the shoulders. Traction will also stretch the brachial plexus of the cervical nerve roots with an Erb's palsy as the potential result (Gordon *et al* 1973; Stevenson *et al* 1982; Spellacy *et al* 1985).

■ Incidence

There is general agreement that the incidence of shoulder dystocia is approximately two per thousand deliveries (0.2 per cent), and that the risk of shoulder dystocia increases with increasing birthweight (Hopwood 1982; Acker *et al* 1986; Gross *et al* 1987a; Al-Najashi *et al* 1989; Vermeulen & Brolmann 1990).

Acker and colleagues (1985) identified infants of non-diabetic mothers with birthweights 4000–4499 g as having a 10 per cent risk of shoulder dystocia while in infants with birthweights >4500 g the risk increased to 22.6 per cent. However infants weighing over 4000 g born to diabetic mothers had a 31 per cent risk of shoulder dystocia. These findings were confirmed by Stevenson *et al* (1982), Boyd *et al* (1983), and Al-Najashi *et al* (1989).

■ Prediction and outcome

Shoulder dystocia usually occurs unexpectedly (Schwartz & McClelland Dixon 1958; Harris 1984; Al-Najashi *et al* 1989; O'Leary & Leonetti 1990). In some cases the first hint of trouble may be slow extension of the baby's head, the chin remaining tight against the mother's perineum.

Benedetti and Gabbe (1978) suggested that a significant decrease in maternal and neonatal morbidity could be achieved if a patient population at risk from shoulder dystocia could be identified. The accurate antenatal diagnosis of the large infant remains a challenge for, as Modanlou (1982) pointed out, the ultrasonic diagnosis of macrosomia (birthweight > 4000g) is not always accurate. The improvement in ultrasonic measurement over a decade has not improved the diagnosis of macrosomia to any significant degree, Chauhan and colleagues (1992) finding that ultrasonic estimation of fetal weight is generally not more accurate than clinical estimation. However, Combs and colleagues (1993) remind us that sonographic estimation of fetal weight is widely used as it is objective and can be reproduced.

O'Leary (1992) concludes that in many circumstances ultrasound gives results that are accurate enough when used with clinical judgment to make a decision about method of delivery. Al-Najashi *et al* (1989) suggest that, to avoid the potentially lethal complications of shoulder dystocia, clinical and technological methods should be used to detect infants of excessive size so that abdominal delivery may be performed.

The diabetic mother and her infant have come under scrutiny by Elliott and colleagues (1982) who found a different body configuration in these infants than the infants of the non-diabetic mother. Increased fat depositions in various organs are thought to be due to insulin secretion in response to maternal hyperglycaemia. Modanlou *et al* (1982) matched a group of babies of diabetic and non-diabetic mothers for weight and gestational age. They found that, even when the mother's diabetes was well controlled, the shoulder and chest sizes in the diabetic group were significantly larger ($p < .005$), although the head circumferences were not significantly different. A study of 70 diabetic pregnancies, (Elliott *et al* 1982 found that in those infants whose chest diameter was 1.4cm or more greater than the biparietal diameter, there was an 87 per cent incidence of shoulder dystocia and concluded that the incidence of traumatic morbidity could be reduced if those infants could be identified and delivered by caesarean section.

As no single test currently establishes the fetus at risk of shoulder dystocia it is advisable to look at all the potential risk factors that may be involved.

☐ Maternal risk factors

Antenatal There are no individually reliable criteria for predicting shoulder dystocia. However, with so many risk factors the problem may be anticipated in some cases. Spellacy and colleagues (1985) found that maternal characteristics for increased risk of delivery of a macrosomic infant, and therefore corresponding risk for shoulder dystocia, were obesity (weight at delivery > 90kg), increased age (over 35), and diabetes mellitus. Smeltzer (1986) more specifically identified the risks of shoulder dystocia complicating delivery. These included maternal obesity (pre-pregnant weight >70kg), multiparity, previous delivery complicated by shoulder dystocia, previous macrosomic infant, and postmaturity (>42 weeks) Maternal obesity is the most frequently occuring factor and is also associated with the highest incidence of shoulder dystocia (Sack 1969; Modanlou *et al* 1982; Boyd *et al* 1983; Acker *et al* 1985; Acker *et al* 1986; Spellacy *et al* 1985).

Klebanoff *et al* (1985) and Seidman *et al* (1988) found that maternal birthweight, especially macrosomia, was an accurate predictor of fetal macrosomia, and went on to suggest that perhaps we should record the mother's own birthweight as part of our obstetric booking history. It should be noted, however, that most factors linked with macrosomia are poor predictors, their presence only serving to *increase* the risk.

A formula for teaching the assessment of the risk of shoulder dystocia was devised by O'Leary (1992: 60) and appears to be used widely in the United States. These risk scores, adapted from the American text (Tables 4.2–4.4) may be used to help to identify those women who may be at risk for shoulder dystocia. The formula allows for women to be reassessed while in labour, taking into account their antenatal score (Table 4.3). The risk of shoulder dystocia complicating a delivery is difficult to assess; this scoring system may prove useful to midwives in practice as an adjunct to their clinical acumen, *not* as a replacement.

Table 4.1 Antenatal risk factors for shoulder dystocia

• Obesity	>70 kg pre-pregnant
	>90 kg at term
• Age	>35
• Multiparity	
• Diabetes mellitus or gestational diabetes	
• History of previous large infant	
• History of previous shoulder dystocia	
• Postmaturity > 42 weeks	

Table 4.2 Antenatal shoulder dystocia risk score

Factor	2	1	0
Estimated fetal weight (kg)	≥4.3	3.8–4.2	<3.8
Maternal weight gain (kg)	>16	12–16	<12
Maternal weight pre-pregnant (kg)	>80	70–80	<70
Glucose intolerance	yes	suspected	no
Gestation (weeks)	>42	41–42	<41

A combined score of 8–10 represents the greatest risk, 4–7 intermediate risk and 0–3 negligible risk
(After O'Leary 1992: 60)

Table 4.3 Intrapartum shoulder dystocia risk score

Factor	2	1	0
Antenatal score	8–10	4–7	0–3
First stage of labour	prolonged latent phase	protracted	normal
Second stage of labour	prolonged	borderline	normal
Birthweight (kg) (estimated)	>4.2	3.8–4.2	<3.8
Forceps delivery	midcavity	low/mid cavity	low

A combined score of 8–10 represents great risk, 4–7 intermediate risk and 0–3 negligable risk
(After O'Leary 1992: 60)

Intrapartum Identifiable risk factors for the intrapartum period found by Benedetti and Gabbe (1978) were: the need for oxytocin augmentation of labour followed by prolonged second stage of labour (>2 hours), then a mid pelvic operative delivery. These factors together with a macrosomic fetus increased the incidence of shoulder dystocia from 1.2 to 23 per cent. O'Leary (1992) agrees that this labour pattern gives warning of shoulder dystocia.

Retrospective analysis of these scoring systems by O'Leary (1992) found that, following vaginal delivery, 17 per cent of the

Table 4.4 Intrapartum risk factors for shoulder dystocia
(Benedetti & Gabbe 1978; O'Leary 1992)

- Macrosomia
- Abnormal first stage of labour
- Oxytocin augmentation of labour
- Prolonged latent phase of labour
- Prolonged second stage of labour with failure or arrest of descent
- The need for mid pelvic forceps delivery

Table 4.5 Shoulder dystocia: potential maternal outcomes

- Postpartum haemorrhage
- Vaginal lacerations
- Uterine rupture
- Third or fourth degree perineal tear
- Vulval haematoma
- Vaginal haematoma
- Cervical tear
- Death

infants born to mothers with high risk scores needed recuscitation when compared with 3 per cent of infants whose mothers had low risk scores.

□ **Potential maternal outcomes**

Maternal injuries following delivery include postpartum haemorrhage; Benedetti and Gabbe (1978) found that 68 per cent of mothers lost over 1000 mls of blood. Other injuries are listed in Table 4.5. In some cases, shoulder dystocia has resulted in maternal death associated with fundal pressure and ruptured uterus and haemorrhage (Kinch 1962; Seigworth 1966; Harris 1984; Al-Najashi *et al* 1989).

If a practitioner believes that a woman in her care is at risk of a delivery being complicated by shoulder dystocia then it would be prudent if the wisdom of delivering in a consultant unit was explained. The choice, however is ultimately the woman's.

Gross *et al* (1987b) conclude that in the pregnancies that result in deliveries of infants of 4000 g or less, the occurrence of shoulder dystocia cannot be predicted from clinical characteristics or labour abnormalities. However if birthweight greater that 4000 g is suspected, then it would be prudent to avoid over zealous attempts at vaginal delivery as this is the apparent cause of most fetal and maternal injury (Boyd *et al* 1983). Potential dangers of vaginal delivery have lead to macrosomia being suggested as a primary indication for caesarean section near term (Parks & Ziel 1978). Since elective surgery is safer than emergency procedures Feldman & Freiman (1985) went even further and suggested prophylactic caesarean section at term could be offered to all. Bromwich (1986) suggests that this approach is unnecessarily radical but if we were aware of the size of fetus before delivery then, perhaps, some maternal and fetal morbidity could be avoided.

☐ Fetal outcomes

William Smellie wrote in 1730:

> A sudden call to a gentlewoman in labour. The child's head delivered for a long time – but even with hard pulling from the midwife, the remarkably large shoulder prevented delivery. I have been called by midwives to many cases of this kind, in which the child is frequently lost.

The outcome for the infant following shoulder dystocia is frequently poor. Consistently authors show that the highest risk of orthopaedic and neurological damage occurs when traction and fundal pressure are used together, (Boyd *et al* 1983; Al-Najashi *et al* 1989; Allen *et al* 1991; O'Leary 1992). Allen *et al* (1991) conducted a series of experiments that showed that during delivery the amount of force applied by the clinician and the duration for which the force was applied more than doubled during a delivery where shoulder dystocia was involved compared with a normal delivery. They used this data to help to predict thresholds for birth injury.

McRoberts' manoeuvre, delivery of the posterior arm and corkscrew manoeuvres appear to be associated with least trauma (Sack 1969; Modanlou *et al* 1980; Boyd *et al* 1983; Spellacy *et al* 1985; Bromwich 1986; Al-Najashi *et al* 1989).

It is obvious that the presence of a person trained in advanced neonatal resuscitation is needed as soon as possible to obtain swift resuscitation and facilitate the best outcome possible.

■ Mechanism and management of shoulder dystocia

In practice, serious difficulty encountered in delivering the shoulders happens when the shoulders try to enter the pelvis in the anterior posterior (narrowest) diameter of the pelvic brim. At term the shoulder or bisacromial diameter is larger than the diameters of the head which have already negotiated the pelvis. Following delivery of the head the posterior shoulder usually slips into the hollow of the sacrum. The anterior shoulder either remains above the pelvic brim, or slips down towards the obturator foramen. When gentle downward traction is applied to the superior aspect of the fetal head and neck, the anterior shoulder either enters the pelvis or rotates from the foramen for delivery.

Shoulder dystocia is characterised by impaction of the anterior shoulder on the symphysis pubis. The posterior shoulder is most distant from the outlet and is therefore under most traction from the neck and the head (Dignam 1976; Hopwood 1982; Smeltzer 1986). Attempts to deliver the anterior shoulder by traction alone at this point will further wedge the anterior shoulder onto the symphysis pubis and further impact the posterior shoulder. Application of inappropriate force tends to impede rather than promote delivery (Gross *et al* 1987a).

Manoeuvres which can be used to persuade the shoulders to negotiate the pelvis so that delivery may be safely completed will now be considered.

● **Before any manoeuvres are attempted an explanation of the problem must be given to the mother and her partner. The co-operation of both will be needed to facilitate a successful outcome.**

□ Manoeuvres involving changing the woman's position

The McRoberts' manoeuvre In 1983 Gonik and colleagues reported a method for the management of shoulder dystocia. The manoeuvre was named after William A McRoberts Jr MD, who had popularised its use in the medical school at Houston Texas. The simplicity of this technique disguises the complex physical and mechanical forces that it invokes.

The manoeuvre involves an exaggerated flexion of the woman's legs into a knee chest position (see Fig. 4.2). Smeltzer (1986) suggests that the McRoberts' manoeuvre causes the anterior shoulder of the fetus to rise free above the mother's symphysis pubis. Thus the whole of the fetus moves anteriorly and the fetal spine

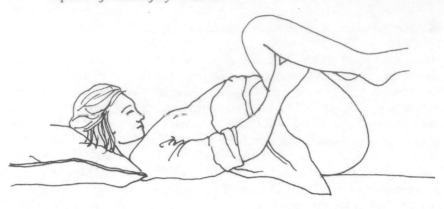

Figure 4.2 Positioning for the McRoberts' manoeuvre

flexes towards the anterior shoulder. The action of lifting and flexion pushes the posterior shoulder over the sacrum through the pelvic inlet. The manoeuvre appears to straighten out the maternal lumber spine; the sacral promontory is removed as an obstruction to the inlet and weightbearing forces are removed from the sacrum, the main pressure point of the pelvis in a lithotomy position (Fig. 4.3a). The symphysis rotates superiorly by about 8 cm, which also brings the plane of the inlet at right angles to the maximum maternal expulsive force (Fig. 4.3b).

There is no claim that the McRoberts' manoeuvre increases the dimensions of the pelvis. It does, however, reverse almost all of the factors causing shoulder dystocia that are created by dorsal and lithotomy positions and to a lesser extent semi recumbent positions. While describing the McRoberts' manoeuvre as 'simple', Smeltzer (1986) points out that it needs no rehearsal.

Gonik and colleagues (1989) used maternal and pelvic models to acquire data on the force needed to extract fetal shoulders. When they compared lithotomy with McRoberts' positioning, there was a consistent reduction in the force needed to extract the fetal shoulders with the latter manoeuvre. The results of this study document objectively that McRoberts' positioning reduces the force needed to extract the shoulders, stretching of the brachial plexus and the incidence of fracture of the clavicle.

O'Leary and Pollack (1991) undertook a survey of 108 hospitals regarding the utilisation and teaching of the McRoberts' manoeuvre amongst obstetricians. Surprisingly only 40 per cent of hospitals taught the manoeuvre but 64 per cent of obstetricians reported being familiar with its use. Amongst users, only 32 per cent used it as an initial step, despite 40 per cent believing

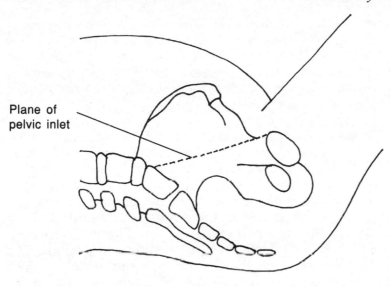

Plane of
pelvic inlet

Figure 4.3a The angle of the pelvis with the woman in dorsal
position (legs in the lithotomy position)

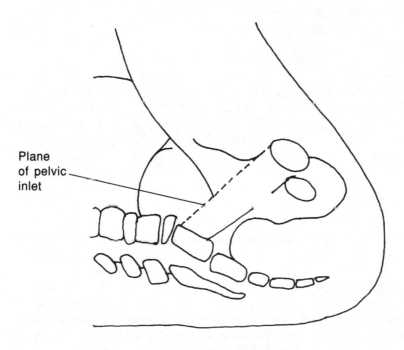

Plane
of pelvic
inlet

Figure 4.3b The angle of the pelvis for McRoberts' manoeuvre

that it reduced the incidence of fetal trauma. However, many authors (Gonik *et al* 1983; Harris 1984; Smeltzer 1986; Gross *et al* 1987a; Mashburn 1988; O'Leary & Pollack 1991) advocate the use of the McRoberts' manoeuvre as a first step once shoulder dystocia has been diagnosed, and suggest that it is worth trying a second time if it fails initially.

All fours position   A minor degree of shoulder dystocia may be alleviated with any movement by the mother, the anterior shoulder is rocked off the symphysis pubis and may then enter the pelvic cavity for completion of delivery. There will be times when the McRoberts' manoeuvre will not be the most appropriate first step to try when faced with shoulder dystocia depending upon where and how the mother has chosen to deliver. The all fours position may be useful as any changes in the mother's position may dislodge the anterior shoulder and alleviate the problem. However a more major problem may not be helped as the health professional is working against gravity. The anterior shoulder could remain caught on the symphysis pubis.

If the mother adopts this position for delivery and chooses to remain in this position, however, then direct manipulation of the fetus may be undertaken (Gaskin 1988; see also the section on Rubin's manoeuvre, below).

□ **Manoeuvres utilising pressure**

Kristeller expression (fundal pressure)   Fundal pressure has been used to supplement expulsive forces (Sandberg 1985). A review of 10 662 vaginal deliveries performed over a five year period in Toronto (Gross *et al* 1987a), revealed that fundal pressure when used without other manoeuvres was associated with a 77 per cent rate of neurological and orthopaedic damage for the fetus. The damage is caused by the impaction of the anterior shoulder onto the symphysis pubis. Fundal pressure necessitates a higher degree of traction to accomplish delivery and is associated with increased risk of injury to the brachial plexus (Schwartz & McClelland Dixon 1958; Dignam 1976; Harris 1984; Gross *et al* 1987a).

Harris (1984), and O'Leary (1992) suggest that fundal pressure may cause uterine rupture and could increase the risk of premature separation of the placenta with the attendant risk of haemorrhage and fetal death. Both authors write that this a rare but possible outcome, but do not elaborate further.

It would appear that fundal pressure is a hazardous procedure with a poor outcome and that it only seems to compound existing problems. Attempting this manoeuvre would delay implementation of more effective techniques (Gross *et al* 1987b). Tolin writes, 'Most cases involving mismanagement of a dystocia delivery involve the impaction of the anterior shoulder against the pubic bone by fundal pressure. . . . experts will testify that it is a deviation from medical standards of care to use fundal pressure' (Tolin 1992: 210).

Suprapubic pressure The aim of using suprapubic pressure is to dislodge the anterior shoulder from the pubic bone to allow it to enter the pelvis and rotate for delivery.

Barnum (1945) warned against the use of suprapubic pressure alone as it may subject the fetal thorax to excessive compression which he felt may lead to cardiac arrest. O'Leary and Pollack (1991), however, suggest that correctly applied suprapubic pressure may be effective. The method advocated is to apply gentle pressure with the palm of the hand, not the fist, on the same side as the fetal back, the pressure directed towards the midline (Fig. 4.4). This in effect will adduct the shoulders and may decrease the bisacromial diameter, allowing the shoulder to rotate off the pubic bone and into the pelvis. This manoeuvre alone is only effective in very mild degrees of dystocia, but has been found to be more effective when used in conjunction with other, usually direct, manoeuvres detailed below.

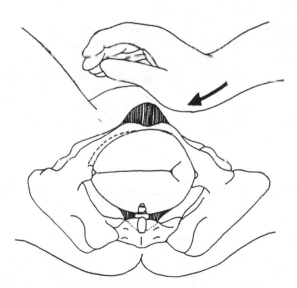

Figure 4.4 Diagram to illustrate the correct use and direction of suprapubic pressure (the fetal back is on the maternal left)

☐ **Manoeuvres requiring direct manipulation of the fetus**

As far as possible analgesia or anaesthesia should be obtained for the mother at this point.

Woods' screw manoeuvre Woods applied the principle of physics to resolve the problem of shoulder dystocia:

> A screw is a continuous spiral on an inclined plane, which when engaged in suitable threads is used to create the greatest resistance to its release by pull.
>
> Woods 1943: 797

Woods demonstrated with a wooden mannikin that, after the head had been born, the shoulders of the baby 'resemble a longitudinal section of a screw engaged in three threads, the pubic thread, the promontory thread and the coccyx thread' (p. 798). Woods went on to state that any pulling on the baby's neck or axilla would be incorrect as it contravenes the laws of physics. The method he used to relieve dystocia was to apply firm but gentle pressure on to the buttocks of the fetus using only the left hand, whilst two fingers of the right hand are used to rotate the shoulders through 180° by exerting pressure onto the anterior surface of the posterior shoulder, the rotation taking place in the direction of the fetal back. Woods claimed that no stretching of the trapezius and no injury of the cervical nerves should occur with this method. The pressure is always directed away from the perineum so trauma to the mother is also minimised.

The manoeuvres that Woods described may have been modified but the principle has been advocated by many (Schwartz & McClelland Dixon 1958; Kinch 1962; Seigworth 1966; Hopwood 1982; Nocon *et al* 1993). The principle remains, 'a direct pull is the most difficult way to release a screw' (Woods 1943).

The Rubin manoeuvre In 1964 Rubin wrote about the importance of bringing both of the shoulders towards the fetal chest, that is adducting the shoulders, to reduce the bisacromial diameter (Fig. 4.5). To achieve this the midwife's hand must be inserted into the vagina and working from behind the fetus should displace the posterior shoulder by pushing the shoulder towards the fetal chest. Rubin also suggests that the anterior shoulder may be rocked by pushing on mother's abdomen from side to side. This may free the anterior shoulder and give the posterior shoulder room to turn. Rubin's methods have been endorsed by other authors since (Dignam 1976; Hopwood 1982; Smeltzer 1986).

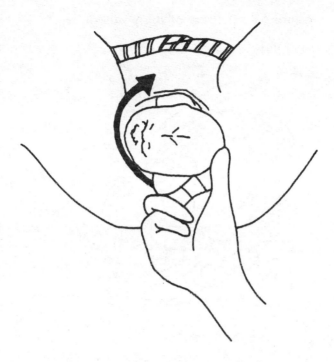

Figure 4.5   Diagram to show the direction of rotation for Rubin's manocuvre when the fetal back is on the maternal left

Delivery of the posterior arm   Barnum (1945) suggested this manoeuvre as an effective method for the relief of shoulder dystocia.

To effect this manoeuvre, insert one hand into the vagina and locate the posterior arm or hand (Fig. 4.6a). The arm should be flexed at the elbow then swept over the chest (Fig. 4.6 b & c). Delivery of the arm is followed by a rotation of the fetus through 180° with the help of an assistant who should push the fetal back over the midline to the other side of the mother's abdomen, (see Fig. 4.4, above).

This manocuvre is said to completely unlock the obstruction by bringing the posterior shoulder under the symphysis pubis, allowing the rest of the body to be born normally.

Schwartz & McClelland Dixon (1958) stated that the extraction of the posterior arm and shoulder were simple and relatively safe compared with traction and pressure. Reporting on a series of 50 cases of shoulder dystocia, traction was used to deliver 31 infants, of whom nine died and seven were 'damaged'. Extraction of the posterior arm was used for the other 19 babies, amongst whom no deaths were recorded. Four of these 19 were 'damaged'.

Figure 4.6 Delivery of the posterior arm

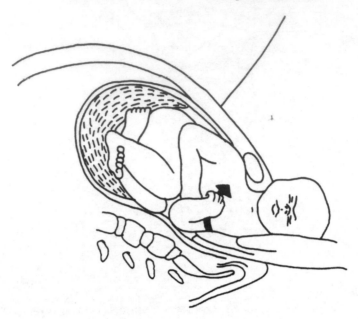

4.6a Locate posterior arm

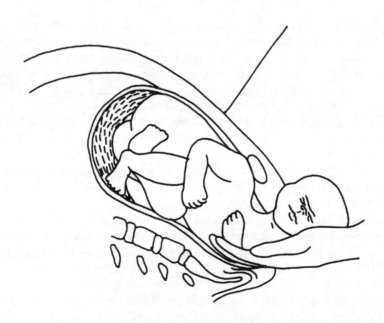

4.6b Grasp arm or hand

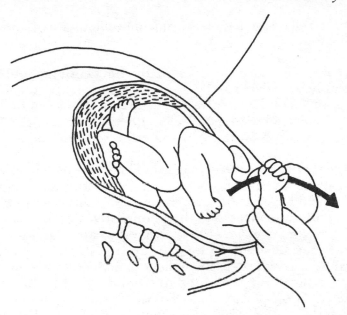

4.6c Deliver the posterior arm by sweeping the arm across the chest

☐ **Surgical procedures**

Fracture of the clavicle and cleidotomy The fracturing of a clavicle is mentioned here as it sometimes happens spontaneously during a delivery complicated by shoulder dystocia, and does not usually produce permanent injury. However, cleidotomy is considered a mutilating and dangerous procedure for both mother and fetus and is a procedure that is now considered to be a destructive operation, and has been described as being almost impossible even in a dead fetus (O'Leary 1992).

Episiotomy Although shoulder dystocia is a bony dystocia not a soft tissue obstruction, episiotomy is recommended by all the authors, with only one exception (Gaskin 1988). An episiotomy gives extra space at the introitus for the clinician to insert a hand past the head and attempt any direct manoeuvres or manipulation. In these circumstances, an episiotomy may protect the mother's perineum and pelvic floor from some further degree of damage.

Performing an episiotomy may be difficult in this situation. Assistance is required at this point to help to (gently) direct the infant's chin away from the perineum during infiltration of local anaesthetic (if the urgency of the situation allows this), and subsequent incision.

Symphysiotomy The surgical division of the symphysis pubis to enlarge the bony pelvis has been practised for many years, and was a relatively safe alternative to caesarean section before the advent of modern anaesthesia. Brews (1948: 763) cites Jean René Sigault as the first physician to have performed the operation in 1777.

Bromwich (1986) suggests that symphysiotomy may help when delivering unexpectedly large shoulders. Only two authors however – Hartfield (1986) and Broekman *et al* (1994) demonstrate the clinical usefulness of symphysiotomy in cases of shoulder dystocia. Broekman *et al* (1994) suggest that, although symphysiotomy may be used to help overcome shoulder dystocia, the procedure carries with it an element of danger for the mother.

Maternal morbidity relating to symphysiotomy (used for cephalopelvic disproportion) was assessed by Broekman and colleagues (1994). In the 1752 cases, problems included 32 cases of pain or other long term difficulties in walking (1.8 per cent), 10 cases of osteitis pubis and retropubic abscess (0.6 per cent), 30 vesicovaginal fistulae (1.7 per cent), and 33 lesions of the anterior wall of the vagina, including the urethra (1.9 per cent). Some women were reported as having more than one problem, though no figure was given for this group.

Thus the literature can be seen to demonstrate that symphysiotomy can be useful in some cases, while highlighting the potential dangers. It is insufficient, however, to assess fully the value of this technique.

The Zavanelli manoeuvre All of the manoeuvres described earlier in this chapter have been directed at completing a safe vaginal delivery. The Zavanelli manoeuvre, however, is a revolutionary concept: replacement of the infant's head into the vagina to be followed by subsequent caesarean section (Sandberg 1985). This manoeuvre and subsequent caesarean delivery was possibly first undertaken by Dr George White in 1945 (cited by Sandberg 1988). The mother, and an infant weighing 15lbs $\frac{1}{2}$ oz, were reported to have made an uneventful recovery. Although Sandberg (1985) suggests that this manoeuvre was conceived out of desperation, O'Leary (1992) states that the technique was developed by Gunn in 1976 in anticipation of the undeliverable shoulder dystocia (reported by O'Leary and Gunn in 1985).

The manoeuvre is carried out thus: the head is manually returned to its pre-restitution position, that is fully extended in a

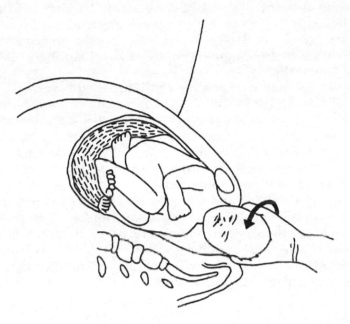

Figure 4.7a Zavanelli manoeuvre: if necessary the head is rotated back to its pre-restitution position

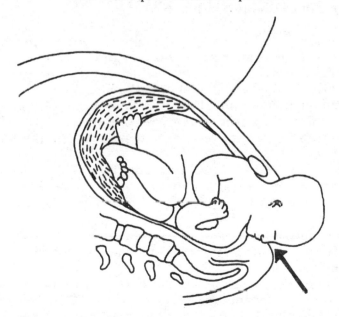

Figure 4.7b Zavanelli manoeuvre: the head is flexed and pushed back into the vagina

direct occipito anterior position (Figure 4.7a). The head is then manually flexed, thus reversing the mechanism for delivery of the head by extension. Upward pressure may be necessary to return the head to the vagina (Figure 4.7b) (Sandberg 1985; O'Leary & Gunn 1985).

In a series of four cases using cardiotocograph recordings, O'Leary and Gunn (1985) found that the infants showed initial bradycardia of 60–70 beats per minute for 2–4 minutes after reinsertion before the heart beat returned to a normal baseline with good variability. It would appear that if the infant has not had any prolonged period of asphyxia prior to the manoeuvre then the experience is well tolerated.

Sandberg (1985; 1988) and Gallaspy *et al* (1991) suggest that, although the Zavanelli manoeuvre is controversial, it is potentially life-saving and therefore deserves to be on every obstetricians' list of salvage techniques. Sandberg (1985) qualifies this by stating that the Zavanelli manoeuvre '. . . must occupy the bottom priority until its virtue and applicability . . . can be confirmed'.

■ Recommendations for clinical practice in the light of currently available evidence

1. Application of O'Leary's antenatal and intrapartum risk scores may help to identify those at risk.
2. Maternity units should have a policy for the recognition and management of dysfunctional labour, and documentation should show that these principles have been followed, (Gross *et al.* 1987b).
3. Accurate intrapartum records may help to identify those at risk.
4. Every unit – and each individual midwife – should have a well-rehearsed plan of action to cope with shoulder dystocia if and when it arises. Such a plan of action could include:
    - Stop pulling;
    - Call for assistance – obstetrician, anaesthetist and paediatrician;
    - If appropriate help the woman into the all fours position;
    - McRoberts' manoeuvre.
5. If the McRoberts' manoeuvre has not been successful in releasing the anterior shoulder then the mother should be left in that position if possible. Otherwise the lithotomy position should be used and the mother's buttocks brought

as far beyond the end of the bed as possible to ensure there is no restriction to the coccyx and sacrum. Whichever of the following manoeuvres are necessary or possible should then be undertaken:

- Episiotomy
- Woods' screw manoeuvre
- Rubin's manoeuvre
- Delivery of the posterior arm

The choice of appropriate manoeuvre should be made by the midwife conducting the case – '. . . no protocol should serve to substitute for clinical judgement' (Nocon *et al.* 1993: 1732).

6. Accurate records of all events must be made as contemporaneously as possible.

■ Practice check

- Do you have a series of manoeuvres that you have committed to memory for a case of shoulder dystocia?
- Do you have useful guidelines for coping with a case of shoulder dystocia on your labour ward?
- If you are unfamiliar with the manoeuvres described in this chapter then perhaps you could practise them using a doll and pelvis.
- Do you ensure that women who have experienced a delivery complicated by shoulder dystocia have time to talk through their experience with a midwife who was present at delivery?
- Do the midwives involved with the delivery have a chance to debrief?
- Do the women who have had a delivery complicated by shoulder dystocia know this fact so that they could inform their midwife or obstetrician in any future pregnancies?
- Are you proficient at resuscitation of the newborn?

☐ **Acknowledgement**

The author wishes to thank Lindsay Keir for producing the illustrations included in this chapter.

■ **References**

Acker DB, Sachs BP, Friedman EA 1985 Risk factors for shoulder dystocia. Obstetrics and Gynecology 66(6): 762–8

Acker DB, Sachs BP, Friedman EA 1986 Risk factors for shoulder dystocia in the average weight infant. Obstetrics and Gynecology 67(5): 614–18

Allen R, Sorab J, Gonik B 1991 Risk factors for shoulder dystocia: an engineering study of clinician-applied forces. Obstetrics and Gynecology 77(3): 352–5

Allott H 1994 A grief shared. British Medical Journal 308:602

Al-Najashi S, Al-Suleiman SA, El-Yahia A, Raman MS, Raman J 1989 Shoulder dystocia – a clinical study of 56 cases. Australian & New Zealand Journal of Obstetrics and Gynecology 29: 129–31

Barnum CG 1945 Dystocia due to the shoulders. American Journal of Obstetrics and Gynecology 50:439–442

Benedetti TJ, Gabbe SG 1978 Shoulder dystocia: a complication of fetal macrosomia and prolonged second stage of labour with mid pelvic delivery. Obstetrics and Gynecology 52(5): 526–9

Bennet CG, Harrold AJ 1976 Prognosis and management of birth injury to the brachial plexus. British Medical Journal 1: 1520–21

Boyd ME, Usher RH, McLean FH 1983 Fetal macrosomia, prediction, risks, proposed management. Obstetrics and Gynecology 61(6): 715–22

Bromwich P 1986 Big babies. British Medical Journal 293: 1387–8

Chemlow D, Kilpatrick SJ, Laros RK 1993 Maternal and neonatal outcomes after prolonged latent phase. Obstetrics and Gynecology 81(4): 486–91

Chauhan SP, Lutton PM, Bailey KJ, Guerrieri JP, Morrison JC 1992 Intrapartum clinical, sonographic, and parous patients' estimates of newborn birth weight. Obstetrics and Gynecology 79: 956–8

Combs CA, Singh NB, Khoury JC 1993 Elective induction versus spontaneous labour after sonographic diagnosis of fetal macrosomia. Obstetrics and Gynecology 81(4): 492–6

Diagnam WJ 1976 Difficulties in delivery, including shoulder dystocia and malpresentations of the fetus. Clinical Obstetrics and Gynecology 19(3): 577–85

Elliott JP, Garite TJ, Freeman RK, McQuown DS, Patl JM 1982 Ultrasonic prediction of fetal macrosomia in diabetic patients. Obstetrics and Gynecology 60(2): 159–62

Feldman GB, Freiman JA 1985 Prophylactic cesarean section at term? New England Journal of Medicine 312(19): 1264–7

Gaskin IM 1988 Shoulder dystocia: controversies in management. Birth Gazette 5(1): 14–17

Gallaspy JW, Dunnihoo DR, DeGueurce JC, Hogan GR, Otterson WN 1991 Cephalic replacement in severe shoulder dystocia. Southern Medical Journal 84(11): 1373–4

Golditch IM, Kirkman K 1978 The large fetus: management and outcome. Obstetrics and Gynecology 52(1): 26–30

Gonik B, Allen Stringer C, Held B 1983 An alternate maneuver for management of shoulder dystocia. American Journal of Obstetrics and Gynecology 145: 882–3

Gonik B, Allen R, Sorab J 1989 Objective evaluation of the shoulder dystocia phenomenon: effect of maternal pelvic orientation on force reduction. Obstetrics and Gynecology 74(1): 44–8

Gordon M, Rich H, Deutschberger G, Green M 1973 Immediate and long term outcome of obstetric birth trauma. American Journal of Obstetrics and Gynecology 117: 51–6

Gross SJ, Shime J, Forrine D 1987a Shoulder dystocia: Predictors and outcome. A five year review. American Journal of Obstetrics and Gynecology 56(2): 334–6

Gross TL, Sokol RJ, Williams T, Thompson K 1987b Shoulder dystocia: a fetal-physician risk. American Journal of Obstetrics and Gynecology 56(6): 1408–18

Harris BA 1984 Shoulder dystocia. Clinical Obstetrics and Gynecology 27(1): 106–11

Hopwood HG 1982 Shoulder dystocia: fifteen years experience in a community hospital. American Journal of Obstetrics and Gynecology 29(2): 162–6

Kinch RAH 1962 Shoulder girdle dystocia. Clinical Obstetrics and Gynecology 5: 1031–43

Klebanoff MA, Mills JL, Berendes HW 1985 Mother's birthweight as a predictor of macrosomia. American Journal of Obstetrics and Gynecology 153: 253–6

Mashburn J 1988 Identification and management of shoulder dystocia. Journal of Nurse-Midwifery 33(5): 225–31

Modanlou HD, Dorchester WL, Thorosian A, Freeman RK 1980 Macrosomia – maternal fetal and neonatal implications. Obstetrics and Gynecology 55(4): 420–24

Modanlou HD, Komatsu G, Dorchester W, Freeman RK, Bosu SK 1982 Large-for-gestational-age neonates: anthropometric reasons for shoulder dystocia. Obstetrics and Gynecology 60(4): 417–23

Morris WIC 1955 Shoulder dystocia. Journal of Obstetrics and Gynaecology of the British Empire 62: 302–6

Nocon JJ, McKenzie DK, Thomas LJ, Hansell RS 1993 Shoulder dystocia: an analysis of risk and obstetric maneuvers. American Journal of Obstetrics and Gynecology 168(6): 1732–9

O'Leary JA, Gunn D 1985 Cephalic replacement for shoulder dystocia. American Journal of Obstetrics and Gynecology 153(3): 592–6

O'Leary JA, Leonetti HB 1990 Shoulder dystocia: prevention and treatment. American Journal of Obstetrics and Gynecology 162(1): 5–9

O'Leary JA, Pollack NB 1991 McRoberts' maneuver for shoulder dystocia: a survey. International Journal of Gynecology and Obstetrics 35(2): 129–31

O'Leary JA 1992 Shoulder dystocia and birth injury: prevention and treatment. McGraw-Hill, New York

Parks DG, Ziel HK 1978 Macrosomia: A proposed indication for primary cesarean section. Obstetrics and Gynecology 52(4): 407–9

Resnik R 1980 Management of shoulder girdle dystocia. Clinical Obstetrics and Gynecology 23(2): 559–64

Rubin A 1964 Management of shoulder dystocia. Journal of the American Medical Association 189: 835

Sack RA 1969 The large infant. American Journal of Obstetrics and Gynecology 104: 195–203

Sandberg EC 1985 The Zavanelli maneuver: a potentially revolutionary method for the resolution of shoulder dystocia. American Journal of Obstetrics and Gynecology 152: 479–84

Sandberg EC 1988 The Zavanelli maneuver extended: progression of a revolutionary concept. American Journal of Obstetrics and Gynecology 158(6): 1347–53

Schwartz BC, McClelland Dixon D 1958 Shoulder dystocia. Obstetrics and Gynecology 11: 468–71

Seidman DS, Ever-Hadani P, Stevenson DK, Slater PE, Harlap S, Gale R 1988 Birth order and birth weight re-examined. Obstetrics and Gynecology 72: 2

Seigworth GR 1966 Shoulder dystocia: review of five years experience. Obstetrics and Gynecology 25(6): 764–7

Smellie W 1730 Treatise on the theory and practice of midwifery Reprinted 1887 McLintock A, (ed) New Sydenham Society, London

Smeltzer JS 1986 Prevention and management of shoulder dystocia. Clinical Obstetrics and Gynecology 29(2): 299–308

Spellacy WN, Miller S, Winegar A, Peterson PQ 1985 Macrosomia – maternal characteristics and infant complications. Obstetrics and Gynecology 66(2): 158–61

Stevenson DK, Hopper AO, Cohen RS, Bucalo LR, Kerner JA, Sunshine P 1982 Macrosomia: causes and consequences. The Journal of Paediatrics 100(4): 515–20

Tolin J 1992 The attorney's viewpoint. In O'Leary JA, (ed) Shoulder dystocia and birth injury: prevention and treatment. McGraw-Hill, New York

Vermeulen GM, Brolmann HA 1990 Shoulder dystocia: a retrospective study. Ned Tijdschr Geneeskd 134(23): 1134–8

Wladimiroff JW, Bloemsma CA, Wallenberg HCS 1978 Ultrasonic diagnosis of the large-for-dates infant. Obstetrics and Gynecology 52(3): 285–7

Woods CE 1943 A principle of physics as applied to shoulder delivery. American Journal of Obstetrics and Gynecology 45: 796–805

Suggested further reading

Allott H 1994 A grief shared. British Medical Journal 308 (6928): 602

Gross SJ, Shime J, Farine D 1987 Shoulder dystocia: predictors and outcome. American Journal of Obstetrics and Gynecology 156(2): 334–6 (MIDIRS Information Pack Number 7 April 1987)

Smeltzer JS 1986 Prevention and management of shoulder dystocia. Clinical Obstetrics and Gynecology 29(2): 299–308

Chapter 5

Drug addicted mothers

Catherine Siney

Drug abuse and pregnancy is not a new phenomenon but it is one that has become more widespread over recent years. For example, prior to 1970 in the New York Downstate Medical Centre the number of infants born to heroin addicted mothers was small (less than 1 in 200) but during the early 1970s these numbers increased to 1 in 69 (Harper *et al* 1974). This trend has continued over subsequent years. Shanley (1986) reported that the numbers of addicted women presenting at a maternity hospital in Sydney had increased from 22 in 1979 to 120 in 1985. Riley (1987) found a dramatic increase at University College Hospital in London; over the previous few years an average of 12 pregnant drug users per year had been seen there, but in 1986, 29 were seen and by the first three months of 1987, 12 had already attended.

In 1988 it was estimated that there were 500 000 heroin addicts in the USA. Of these, approximately 200 000 were women, and at least 5000 babies were born to them every year (Edelin *et al* 1988). The United Kingdom Home Office (cited in Gerada *et al* 1990) estimated that there were between 35 000 and 75 000 notified injecting opiate users; one third were women of whom 80 per cent were of childbearing age. Therefore, in the UK there were between 9000 and 20 000 female notified injecting opiate users of childbearing age.

Inadequate antenatal care has been cited as contributing to the problems experienced by drug using women. For example, a retrospective analysis of the outcomes of approximately 24 000 deliveries taking place between 1983 and 1990 in the USA revealed that drug abusers receiving adequate antenatal care had a 2–3 times higher incidence of low birthweight and perinatal death. When antenatal care was inadequate this rose to a three times incidence of both (Broekhuizen *et al* 1992). These findings emphasise the importance of antenatal (and therefore midwifery) care, in reducing or minimising the problems experienced by these women and their babies.

This chapter outlines the risks to the mother and her baby of drug abuse, traces the management of pregnant drug users over the last 25 years, and describes some of the recent initiatives in helping to reduce the risks of drug abuse in these women. Much of the literature concerns pregnant women addicted to opiates, such as heroin and pethidine, but other groups of drugs – such as cocaine, 'crack' (cocaine in smokeable form), amphetamines, and 'soft' drugs for example cannabis, – are also abused, and many women are polydrug users (Riley 1987). It should be remembered that the lifestyles of many female drug abusers may expose them to poverty, homelessness, poor housing conditions, prostitution, sexual and physical abuse, depression and infections including hepatitis and HIV. For more information on HIV in pregnancy the reader is referred to the chapter in this volume by Carolyn Roth.

■ **It is assumed that you are already aware of the following:**

● The commonly accepted effects of drugs of addiction on the fetus;
● The legal position regarding fetal and maternal rights.

■ **Drug abusing mothers: what are their problems?**

Drug abusing women and their babies are at higher obstetric risk than non-drug abusing women in a number of ways. There is some evidence to suggest that risks can be minimised if women can be identified and given adequate antenatal care (Broekhuizen *et al* 1992; Siney *et al* 1995).

□ **Risks to the mother**

Medical problems Medical problems associated with heavy drug use include malnutrition leading to vitamin deficiencies and anaemia (Riley 1987; Gerada *et al* 1990; Hepburn 1993), chronic bronchitis (Riley 1987) from inhalation of drugs mixed with tobacco (the chapter is not concerned with tobacco addiction, only as a vehicle for other drugs, such as cannabis, heroin or 'crack'), urinary tract infections and sexually transmitted diseases (Riley 1987; Gerada *et al* 1990; Lam 1992; Hepburn 1993) and ante-partum haemorrhage (Gerada *et al* 1990; Lam 1992).

Problems primarily associated with injecting drugs or sharing injecting equipment are hepatitis B, hepatitis C, HIV/AIDS, thrombophlebitis, gangrene, abscesses and septicaemia (Gerada *et al* 1990; HMSO 1991; ISDD 1992).

Social problems Over 20 years ago, the effectiveness of health services as far as individuals from deprived social groups were concerned was seriously questioned (Tudor Hart 1971). More recent authors feel little has changed (Whitehead 1988; Hepburn 1993). Furthermore, there is a close correlation between the use of ilicit drugs and socioeconomic deprivation (Standing Committee on Drug Abuse 1985).

Many drug using mothers are immature and vulnerable to psychiatric problems (Riley 1987). The chaotic lifestyle that may develop as their dependence on illegal substances grows, serves only to increase this vulnerability (Riley 1987).

Observation of pregnant drug addicts in Glasgow led one author to suggest that 'Poor pregnancy outcome in women drug users may be due not so much to the drugs as to the underlying socioeconomic deprivation or the effect of drug use on lifestyle' (Hepburn 1993).

□ Risks to the fetus and neonate

The risks to the fetus if the mother abuses drugs are impairment of development, function and/or growth. A major problem for the fetus is that, whereas the mother can excrete drugs, the fetus cannot do so with the same efficiency and drug levels can accumulate. In general, regardless of the drug taken there is an increased risk of preterm delivery, intrauterine growth retardation and congenital abnormalities with a consequently higher rate of perinatal and infant mortality (Riley 1987; Gerada *et al* 1990; Lam 1992; Dawe *et al* 1992). There are difficulties however with fetal damage studies including extrapolation from animal studies, and the chance of inaccurate history taking of women regarding their true drug habit/intake (Hepburn 1993; Klein *et al* 1993). This often makes it difficult to assess with any degree of accuracy how the drug habits of the mother may affect the fetus.

Lam (1992) found an increased incidence of preterm delivery

and growth retardation (the mean birthweight of babies born to drug abusing mothers was 629 g lighter than those born to non-drug abusing mothers). Dawe and colleagues (1992) reported that 10 of 34 babies were growth-retarded.

□ Identifying risk

The pregnant woman who is using drugs may not reveal this to her midwife or to her health professional (Klein *et al* 1993). There are a number of reasons for this, the two main ones being fear that social services will take their children away and the perceived lack of confidentiality (Gerada *et al*; Hepburn 1993). These problems have meant that it has taken a great deal of time for good communications to build up between drug services and maternity services. Consequently, services that are useful for maintaining healthy pregnancy and good outcome, and which are attractive to the women who may need them, have been slow to develop. The following section of the chapter traces the development and outcomes of these services.

■ Identifying and managing the problems: the past 25 years

In the early 1970s a programme of family and maternity care was organised in New York to try to prevent the multiple medical and social problems associated with addiction and pregnancy (Harper *et al* 1974). A methadone programme was provided, together with help with financial, legal and housing problems. The programme's long term treatment goal was to use pregnancy as an opportunity to motivate a change of lifestyle on the part of the woman or couple. The woman received the same obstetric care (including analgesia) as non addicted women.

Treatment of infant withdrawal symptoms was based upon the infant's clinical condition. Of the 62 women who were followed through their pregnancies and afterwards, 7 (11 per cent) miscarried or had terminations of pregnancy, 51 (83 per cent) delivered liveborn infants and 4 (6 per cent) had stillbirths. Three infants subsequently died; one from cytomegalovirus probably acquired *in utero*, one from bronchopneumonia, and one from diaphragmatic hernia. The conclusions drawn at the end of the first year of the programme was that many of the common maternal problems associated with addiction had been alleviated.

Fraser (1983) conducted a retrospective study in London of 72 pregnancies occurring between 1966 and 1982 to women addicted to methadone and/or heroin, pethidine, or 'soft' drugs. Few of these women received what was considered to be adequate antenatal care, and attempts to admit these women for fetal assessment and drug supervision were largely unsuccessful due to lack of patient co-operation. One of the main problems encountered was accurately assessing the period of gestation, either because the woman could not recall the date of her last menstrual period, or because of amenorrhoea before pregnancy. Eight (11 per cent) of the women stopped drug use during pregnancy. Eleven (15 per cent) required admission antenatally for problems such as pyelonephritis, femoral thrombosis, hepatitis, lung abscess, labial abscess, severe folate deficiency, or following assault. Fourteen (19 per cent) miscarried or had terminations of pregnancy (one illegally, resulting in the death of the mother), and 58 (81 per cent) delivered live infants. There were two perinatal deaths (3 per cent): one for no apparent cause and one due to prematurity. There were no drug related problems with regard to labour and the puerperium. Fraser concluded that the management of pregnancy in drug addicted women was complex, involving medical and social problems before and after pregnancy. He recommended that case conferences should be held as early as possible in these pregnancies to identify and resolve these problems. This study highlighted the problems of identifying drug addicted women and keeping them within the antenatal and social services systems. Fraser recommended that all infants of drug-addicted mothers should be admitted to a special care baby unit for observation for the first week of life and that once symptomatic they should be sedated and the sedation then withdrawn in a controlled manner.

Strang and Moran (1985) of the Manchester Regional Drug Dependence Unit, stressed the importance of a programme of antenatal care which included help to enable the woman to reduce the dosage of her drug of dependence. Following the guidelines of the Medical Working Group on Drug Dependence (1984) they recommended switching the women onto a long-acting orally available drug from the same pharmacological group as the drug of dependence (for example, methadone for heroin). This minimised the likelihood of peaks and troughs in drug circulating levels, and facilitated a gradual reduction in dosage over a period of months. The drug was to be given in divided doses during the day, and regular urine testing undertaken to check compliance. They also recommended that infants who showed opiate withdrawal symptoms should be given opiates and weaned off, but (contrary to previous recommended practice) no sedatives. In the case of maternal barbiturate addiction they recommended the infant should be treated with phenobarbitone, and in the case of maternal benzodiazepine addiction, diazepam. The babies were to be weaned off the treatment slowly, and not breastfed if the mother was still taking the drug of addiction.

Klenka (1986) retrospectively assessed the outcomes of the 25 pregnancies of 23 drug addicted women from Merseyside. All the women were addicted to heroin and some were also addicted to other narcotics or 'soft' drugs. Eight of these women stopped taking drugs during pregnancy, and another eight attempted to stop but were unsuccessful. All the women were referred to a consultant obstetrician for hospital care, and continuity was maintained with the help of the community midwives. All attended the antenatal clinic prior to delivery, but most did not attend until late in their pregnancy. The 25 babies were admitted to the SCBU for observation, and 19 developed withdrawal symptoms within 24–48 hours. Twelve required treatment with phenobarbitone, chloral hydrate, and/or chlorpromazine.

Several programmes of methadone stabilisation and management were instituted (e.g. Strang & Moran 1985; Shanley 1986), but towards the end of the 1980s their efficacy was questioned. Edelin *et al* (1988) reported an analysis of 26 narcotic addicted women who were enrolled in a methadone programme in Massachusetts, USA. These were compared with a similar group of 37 polydrug users not in a methadone programme, and also with a control group of 716 non-drug using pregnant women. When the two drug using groups were compared there was no difference in birthweight or Apgar scores. The only differences noted were that the women in the methadone group made more antenatal visits and had more antenatal care, and experienced less anaemia. When these drug using groups were compared with the non-drug using group, the mean birthweight was higher in the latter (the control group) though the differences were 'not statistically significant'. The results of this study questioned the effectiveness of the methadone programme in promoting fetal growth and wellbeing.

Concerns have been expressed on many occasions (e.g. Edelin 1988; Green & Gossop 1988) that infants born to drug using mothers are exposed to poor mothering and poor environments. Strang and Moran (1985) stressed, however, that parenting skills should be judged by the same criteria applied to non-addicted parents.

Following a study of 12 pregnant opiate users attending the Drug Dependence Unit at the Bethlem Hospital, Green and Gossop (1988) recommended that a key social worker should be appointed early, that these women should be treated as medically high risk, that there should be improved communication between caring agencies and that the mothering skills of drug addicted women should be studied.

The emphasis of management of a pregnant drug user over the years appears to have focused upon protecting the fetus and influencing women to change their lifestyles. Such management programmes can often become judgemental and paternalistic, removing the locus of power and control from drug abusing women and reinforcing feelings of loss of control and low self-esteem.

The role of professionals in pregnancy and childbirth should be to provide information and choice to women, via a supportive service that is easily accessible in order to give back to them power and control over their bodies and lifestyles (Expert Maternity Group 1993). Some maternity services have now recognised the need to involve pregnant drug misusers in the planning of their care and are trying to bring these women back into the mainstream of caring services. The midwife can be pivotal in generating an atmosphere of trust and continuity with the pregnant woman and is the vital link in sharing information with other professionals involved in the care (Latchem 1994; Siney 1994). The next section of this chapter describes the initiatives developed in the 1990s and makes recommendations for the care of drug abusing pregnant women and their babies.

■ Into the 1990s

A group of professionals from the Institute of Psychiatry in London set up a programme to identify drug abusing pregnant women, and to attract them towards the service they offered (Gerada *et al* 1990). This comprised a multidisciplinary approach to providing antenatal and general health care, and help in stabilising and reducing opioid use with the help of a carefully supervised methadone programme. Gerada and colleagues emphasised that drug abuse did not preclude good parenting skills and recommended that these should be assessed independently of the drug habit. They also stressed the importance of providing opportunities to talk about health issues at a time when women were generally compliant because they cared about the pregnancy, and noted that any automatic institution of child care proceedings might be counterproductive, by deterring drug abusing parents from approaching health care professionals.

Breen (1991) also advocated a multidisciplinary approach to drug using women, naming the drug dependency worker, obstetric social worker, health visitor, community midwife, probation officer, district social worker and the GP as members of the team who would meet regularly throughout the pregnancy. Campbell (1990/91) described the management of drug addicted women at the West London Hospital. Like Strang and Moran (1985), Dixon (1987) and Gerada *et al* (1990), Campbell recommended that mothers should be given a chance to prove their parenting skills and argued against judgemental or disapproving attitudes by health care professionals, stressing the importance of considering each case individually. She further recommended that the management of pregnancy should be flexible and that sudden withdrawal of opiates from the mother should be avoided. Labour and delivery should take place in a specialist unit. Campbell pointed out that a paediatrician should be present at delivery and the baby would probably require observation for withdrawal symptoms in a special care baby unit. Withdrawal symptoms would commonly be treated by chlorpromazine.

Partly in order to investigate whether the birth of a baby was sufficient stimulus for the mother to stop drug using, Fraser updated his retrospective study in London of 111 births (including three sets of twins) in 94 women, occurring between 1966 and 1988. The progress of 86 of these women was traceable up to one year was following delivery. Twenty (24 per cent) of the 86 had stopped using drugs. Of the 22 children born to these women, only one was no longer with the mother. Sixty-six women (76 per cent) were still taking drugs, and of the 84 children born to these women 53 (66 per cent) were no longer with the mother. Twenty were adopted, five were in care, five were fostered, six had died and seventeen were with the father or other relatives. The conclusion drawn was that if a mother was successful in stopping drug abuse then she and the child were more likely to remain together (Fraser & Cavanagh 1991).

■ Current initiatives

Dawe and colleagues (1992) discussed the importance of providing a pregnancy liaison and outreach service for female drug users. Hepburn (1993) examined the problems of drug misuse in the context of other severe social problems and advocated an holistic, multidisciplinary, non-judgemental approach to caring for these women. She considered that obstetric management need be little different from the normal routine, although it should reflect the many problems, including social ones, experienced by drug using women.

These themes of multidisciplinary, non-judgemental approaches are reflected in the descriptions below of two different initiatives.

☐ **Liaison Antenatal Drug Service (Latchem 1994)**

The Liaison Antenatal Drug Service (LANDS) at Guy's Hospital, London was set up four years ago. A clinic is held in the hospital preceded by a clinical meeting where members of the multidisciplinary team can exchange information. The team consists of the antenatal midwifery manager, a midwife who rotates between the wards and the antenatal clinic, the liaison health visitor, drug workers from local agencies and a psychiatric senior registrar from the local drug agency. Obstetric and psychiatric consultants are medically responsible for clients and are available for support and advice. An evaluation is currently being undertaken, although the numbers of women involved are too small for critical statistical analysis, many positive improvements in providing care have been identified. For example, amongst regular attendees, there has been a reduction in withdrawal symptoms in the newborn. Babies were less likely to be admitted to the SCBU, had increased birthweight and longer gestation at delivery. Mothers who attended regularly were less likely to have social work intervention than irregular attenders. The increased level of communication with other agencies has given women the opportunity of a healthy birth experience and awareness of support agencies.

☐ **A co-ordinated programme at Liverpool, UK (Siney 1994; Siney *et al* 1995)**

The maternity and gynaecology service developed at the Liverpool Women's Hospital (formerly the Liverpool Maternity Hospital, Mill Road Maternity Hospital and the Women's Hospital), has also reflected the need to look at drug using women in a holistic way and not just as a collection of problems (Siney 1994). It emphasises communication not only between hospital services and agencies working with drug misusers but also between mothers, midwives and doctors. History taking at the hospital asks about past or current use in a non-judgemental way and women are asked if they would like to meet the specialist midwife for advice and/or support. Both midwifery and obstetric staff had discussed how important it was for women to be able to admit drug misuse so that they would be able to ask questions about both their care and the possible effects of drugs on their babies. Two-way communication enables health care professionals to give accurate relevant advice to women and in turn enables women to make decisions and choices. The antenatal care offered to drug using women is no different from that offered to non-drug using women but it is available on both a regular basis at the local drug dependency unit and an *ad hoc* basis at any other site on request, as well as within the antenatal clinic. Regular informal review of all women known to the service takes place, with their knowledge, in the hospital social work department – information being gathered from all agencies caring for or working with the women. Any childcare and other problems foreseen are dealt with before delivery. This allows the women to labour, deliver and be transferred home in the same way as non-drug using women.

Siney and colleagues (1995) compared the outcomes of 103 women (delivered over a 31 month period) on a methadone programme who received regular antenatal care with a matched control group of non-drug using women. This then allowed the writing of guidelines for the management of their pregnancies and the treatment of their infants (Siney, in press). A non-subjective neonatal opiate withdrawal chart was also designed. This chart was audited in 1994 and a new chart was designed (Figure 5.1).

The aim of the service was to 'normalise' the management and attract the women into mainstream care. Between March 1990 to December 1993, 287 pregnant women were referred to the service. Forty-two had miscarriages or terminations of pregnancies. Five women were found not to be pregnant, and there were two intrauterine deaths. Of the remaining women, 220 had live births at the Liverpool Women's Hospital. The specialist midwife acts as a link or liaison for anyone working with pregnant drug misusers.

Study results showed that if women were on a methadone programme, with the support that this entails from drug dependency units, other drug agencies or general practitioners, and they also received regular antenatal care, then the outcomes of pregnancy were as good as similar non-drug misusing women.

LIVERPOOL NEONATAL DRUG WITHDRAWAL CHART

NAME:_____ Casenote No: _____ D.O.B. _____ Gestation: _____

Minor symptoms need not be recorded. If infant unwell or not feeding commence 4 hourly observation for severe symptoms. (Minor symptoms listed for differentiation purpose – tremors when disturbed, respirations > 60 per minute, pyrexia of unknown origin, sweating, frequent yawning, sneezing/nasal stuffiness, poor feeding/regurgitation, loose stools) if treatment of the 3 severe symptoms not judged clinically necessary, then reasons must be recorded in casenotes *Treatment:* 0.125mgs morphine sulphate orally (dependent on body weight) 1st day of treatment – 4 hourly, 2nd – 6 hourly, 3rd-8 hourly 4th – 12 hourly, 5th – daily. Treatment can be commenced at any level and frequency of administration is reduced when asymptomatic for 24 hours. If symptomatic do not reduce level.

Severe symptoms – please tick (✓) if present.

	Date: Time:								
1. Convulsions									

2. Tremors when undisturbed
   Non-stop high pitched cry
   Sleeps<1 hr after good feed									

3. Watery stools projectile vomiting									
Signature:									

	Date: Time:								
1. Convulsions									

2. Tremors when undisturbed
   Non-stop high pitched cry
   Sleeps<1 hr after good feed									

3. Watery stools projectile vomiting									
Signature:									

	Date: Time:								
1. Convulsions									

2. Tremors when undisturbed
   Non-stop high pitched cry
   Sleeps<1 hr after good feed									

3. Watery stools projectile vomiting									
Signature:									

Figure 5.1 Post-audit neonatal drug withdrawal chart

☐ **The role of the midwife**

It is to be hoped that the future of maternity services for drug misusing women and their families will be co-ordinated, putting the woman and her family at the centre, offering her both confidentiality and support. This requires a link professional within the maternity service, preferably a midwife, to liaise with all agencies who care for drug misusers. This midwife should ensure that antenatal care is given, informal social assessment undertaken and any decisions made or case conferences held before the delivery of the infant.

The importance of the midwife's role in caring for drug misusing women cannot be over-emphasised. She has both an educational and a supportive role with pregnant women and it is important that the midwife/client relationship is established to dispel anxiety. The midwife is the link for the women and their families to the maternity services and it is essential that all midwives are given information about the effects of drug misusing on both mother and baby. This should be part of the curriculum for student midwives and form part of continuing education programmes for qualified midwives. If midwives are knowledgeable about the effects of drug misuse on pregnant women and their families then they are enabled to give non-judgemental and supportive care and advice.

This kind of service provision will go some way towards giving these women a positive birth experience.

■ **Recommendations for clinical practice based on currently available evidence**

1. Every effort should be made to gain the trust of the women by offering a service that is both confidential and non-judgemental. Reassurance, encouragement and support should be given to the woman and her partner or family to prepare her for parenting her child.
2. Guidelines for the management of pregnancy and care of neonates should be designed, and all staff should be aware of them. These guidelines should be shared with drug agencies, social service and probation departments.
3. There must be communication, via a link midwife, between drug prescribing agencies/general practitioners and services providing maternity and gynaecology care.
4. Informal assessment of social problems should happen on

a regular basis throughout the pregnancy so that the woman, her family and anyone who is caring for her, know of any problems that occur and can deal with them before the baby is born.

5. Efforts should be made to provide antenatal care at sites that are acceptable and accessible to drug using women.
6. Entry to methadone maintenance/reduction programmes should be available to all pregnant women as a priority.

■ Practice check

- Are you aware of a problem of drug dependency in your area? What sort of communication do you as a midwife have with the drug services?
- What are the formal policies for communicating with your local social services department about individual women? How do these affect confidentiality? Are drug misusers referred to district social service departments automatically?
- How confident are you that your behaviour towards drug using women is sensitive, supportive and non-judgemental? Are you able to discuss this issue with a trusted colleague?
- How would you advise a colleague with no previous experience of pregnant drug users to plan optimal care for such a woman?
- Are known or suspected drug misusers automatically offered HIV or hepatitis B testing? Is there pre-test counselling and support available?
- Does your unit use a neonatal drug withdrawal chart? How subjective is it? How helpful would it be to a midwife with no previous experience of caring for the babies of drug misusers?
- How are the parenting skills of new mothers assessed on the postnatal wards in your unit? Are drug using mothers assessed in the same way? If not, why not?

■ References

Breen M 1991 Treating drug dependency. Nursing Times   87(9): 62–3

Broekhuizen FF, Utrie J, Van Mullem C 1992 Drug use or inadequate prenatal care? Adverse pregnancy outcome in an urban setting. American Journal of Obstetrics and Gynecology 166(6): 1747–56

Campbell MJ 1990/91 Heroin-misuse in pregnancy. Journal of the Association of Chartered Physiotherapists in Obstetrics and Gynecology 68 (Winter): 13–15

Dawe S, Gerada C, Strang J, 1992 Establishment of a liaison service for pregnant opiate-dependent women. British Journal of Addiction 87(6): 867–71

Dixon A 1987 The pregnant addict. Druglink July/August: 6–8

Edelin KC, Gurganious L, Golar K, Oellerich D, Kyei-Aboagye K, Adel-Hamid M 1988 Methadone maintenance in pregnancy: consequences to care and outcome. Obstetrics and Gynecology 71(3): 399–404

Expert Maternity Group 1993 Changing childbirth. HMSO, London

Fraser AC, 1983 The pregnant drug addict. Maternal and Child Health. November: 461–3

Fraser AC, Cavanagh S 1991 Pregnancy and drug addiction – long term consequences. Journal of the Royal Society of Medicine 84(9): 530–32

Gerada C, Dawe S, Farrell M 1990 Management of the pregnant opiate user. British Journal of Hospital Medicine 43(February): 138–41

Green L, Gossop M 1988 The management of pregnancy in opiate addicts. Journal of Reproductive and Infant Psychology 6(1): 51–7

Harper RG, Solish GI, Purow HM, Sang E, Panepinto WC 1974 The effect of a methadone treatment program upon heroin addicts and their newborn infants. Pediatrics 54(3): 300–5

HMSO 1991 Drug misuse and dependence. Guidelines on clinical management: 10. HMSO, London

Hepburn M 1993, Drug use in pregnancy. British Journal of Hospital Medicine 49: 51–5

Institute for the Study of Drug Dependence 1992 Drugs, pregnancy and childcare. A guide for professionals. ISDD, London

Klein RF, Friedman-Campbell M, Tocco RV 1993 History taking and substance abuse counseling with the pregnant patient. Clinical Obstetrics and Gynecology 36(2): 338–46

Klenka HM 1986 Babies born in a district general hospital to mothers taking heroin. British Medical Journal 293: 745–6

Lam SK, To WK, Duthie SJ, Ma HK 1992 Narcotic addiction in pregnancy with adverse maternal and perinatal outcome. Australia & New Zealand Journal of Obstetrics and Gynecology 32(3): 216

Latchem S 1994 Antenatal care for drug users. Health Professional Digest 5: 2–5

Medical Working Group on Drug Dependence 1984 Guidelines. Available from ISDD, London

Riley D 1987 The management of the pregnant drug addict. Bulletin of the Royal College of Psychiatrists 11 (November): 362–4

Shanley C 1986 The management of narcotic dependent pregnancy. Australian Nurses Journal 16 (2): 50–51

Siney C 1994 Team effort helps pregnant drug users. Modern Midwife 4(2): 23–4

Siney C In press Drug misuse and pregnancy. In Karger I (ed) Challenges for midwifery practice. Macmillan, Basingstoke

Siney C, Kidd M, Walkinshaw S, Morrison C, Manasse P 1995 Outcome of pregnancy in opiate dependent women within a methadone treatment programme. British Journal of Midwifery 3 (2): 69–73

Standing Committee on Drug Abuse 1985 Drug problems in greater Glasgow: report of the SCODA Fieldwork survey in Greater Glasgow Health Board. Chameleon Press, London

Strang J, Moran C 1985 The pregnant drug addict. (Unpublished)

Tudor Hart J 1971 The inverse care law. Lancet i: 405–12

Whitehead M 1988 The health divide. Pelican, London

■ Suggested further reading

Institute for the Study of Drug Dependence 1992 Drugs, pregnancy and childcare. A guide for professionals. ISDD, London

HMSO 1991 Drug misuse and dependence. Guidelines on clinical management. HMSO, London

Chapter 6

HIV and pregnancy

Carolyn Roth

The epidemic of infection with Human Immunodeficiency Virus (HIV) and Acquired Immune Deficiency Syndrome (AIDS) to which it leads has had enormous impact on women and babies worldwide. The World Health Organisation (WHO) estimates that in the 13 years since the transmission of Human Immunodeficiency Virus Type 1 (HIV-1) from a mother to her child was first reported (Rogers *et al* 1987), there have been about 500 000 cases of AIDS in women and children worldwide, most of which have been unrecognised (Chin 1990). By early 1990, the WHO estimated that more than three million women, most of child bearing age, were infected with HIV, about 80 per cent of whom were in sub-Saharan Africa. It has been suggested that during the 1990s an additional three million women and children world wide will die as a consequence of the epidemic (Chin 1990).

Heterosexual transmission of HIV is now the fastest growing category of transmission, with women the fastest growing group affected by the epidemic (Bardequez & Johnson 1994), and AIDS has become the leading cause of death for women aged 20–40 in New York as well as most central African cities (Chin 1990).

With the inexorable spread of HIV infection worldwide, has come a growing recognition that its physical, social, economic and demographic impact on women and children has been insufficiently addressed in research and policy discussion (Chin 1990; Hankins 1990; Scharf 1992; Berer 1993).

The model for the definition of AIDS and information on its natural history is derived from the study of gay, largely white and middle class men in developed countries and men with haemophilia (Bardequez & Johnson 1994). There is much less information about the natural history of HIV infection in women, especially non-pregnant women (Bardequez & Johnson 1994). Women have been excluded from, or under represented in trials of antiviral treatment; non-pregnant women have had to meet contraceptive criteria not demanded of men, and it is suspected that women have been considered unreliable and unlikely to comply with contraceptive measures and clinical trial protocols (Hankins 1990: 445; Scharf 1992: 189). The recently reported Concorde trial, comparing the early and late use of zidovudine (Concorde Coordinating Committee 1994), for example, excluded pregnant women. The irony of this has been noted by one observer (Lipsky 1994), as this may have been a group most likely to have benefited from the study, in the light of recent reports (Morbidity & Mortality Report 1994) which suggest the value of zidovudine in reducing perinatal transmission of HIV.

The distribution and impact of HIV infection globally affects populations which vary greatly in relation to socioeconomic circumstances, gender, sexuality and background health circumstances, all of which will influence the pattern of disease associated with immune compromise as well as determine the appropriateness and efficacy of preventive and therapeutic interventions. Hankins (1990) notes that, worldwide, those women most at risk of HIV infection are disadvantaged, disenfranchised and discriminated against in many facets of their lives. The inequalities and lack of social power which women suffer contribute to their vulnerability to HIV infection and exacerbate the profound impact that it has on their lives.

Midwives, as key providers of services to women during pregnancy and childbirth, are well placed both as a source of information about pregnancy and other health issues and to safeguard women's access to choice and control over their care during pregnancy, which is acknowledged to be their entitlement (HC Health Committee 1992; Expert Maternity Group 1993). Midwives are in a favoured position to ensure appropriate responses to women's expressed needs and preferences during pregnancy and childbirth and can make an invaluable contribution to the quality of experience at this time which is liable to be a particularly difficult one for the woman with HIV infection.

This chapter reviews some of the recent research into HIV and pregnancy and highlights some of the issues that are important for midwives' consideration, relating to the care and information which they provide and also to their understanding of the significance of HIV infection for the health of mothers and babies. An attempt has been made not to repeat material already published in this series (Roth & Brierley 1990), and therefore reading this chapter in conjunction with the earlier one is recommended. In addition, because the chapter in this volume by Catherine Siney directly addresses the specific needs of drug dependent women during pregnancy, this chapter does not address that issue.

It is recognised that there are at least two varieties of HIV, designated as HIV-1 and HIV-2. So far, in the UK, HIV-1 is the predominant form and the following discussion relates to HIV-1 unless otherwise stated.

■ It is assumed that you are already aware of the following:

- The characteristics of the Human Immunodeficiency Virus;
- Its modes of transmission;
- Its physical effects;
- The social and psychological implications of being HIV positive;
- Principles of infection control in the health care setting (see Pratt 1992 for background to these issues);
- The particular concerns, for women and professionals, relating to HIV infection during pregnancy (see Roth & Brierley 1990).

■ Current information about HIV in pregnancy

□ Prevalence of HIV amongst pregnant women in Great Britain

There are two sources of information about the prevalence of HIV amongst the pregnant population. Since January 1990, unlinked anonymous seroprevalence monitoring has been carried out based on a number of different population groups, including women attending antenatal clinics. The figures (Table 6.1) demonstrate a much higher prevalence of HIV in London compared with samples from elsewhere in England and Wales.

The National Study of HIV in Pregnancy collates confidential notifications from obstetricians, paediatricians and laboratories, of pregnancies to women known to be HIV positive. A total of 695 pregnancies have been notified from June 1989 to May 1994 (RCOG 1994). The regional breakdown of these pregnancies is illustrated in Table 6.2, and similarly shows a concentration of seropositive women in the London area as well as in Scotland.

Table 6.1   Unlinked anonymous HIV seroprevalence in England
and Wales (PHLS 1993)

Year	Antenatal specimens London (number)	Outside London (number)
1990	0.18% (78)	0.01% (4)
1991	0.22% (118)	0.02% (16)
1992*	0.24% (61)	0.01% (3)

*Data included up to June 1992. Not all centres or districts partici-
pated throughout the period

In their analysis of the epidemiology of vertically acquired
HIV infection (transmission from mother to baby), Ades *et al*
(1993) report that in Scotland and the Irish Republic, where
most HIV infection is associated with intravenous drug use (IVDU)
by the woman or her sexual partner, there has been a fall in
reports of children born to infected mothers since 1989. In England and Wales, approximately half of maternal infection has
been acquired overseas through heterosexual contact and the
number of babies born to this group of women and to women
who have acquired their infection in Britain is increasing.

The study also identified differences in the proportion of
women who are known by the obstetrician to be seropositive before
delivery, which was 68 per cent in Scotland and only 17.4 per
cent in south east England (Ades *et al* 1993). These differences
reflect different approaches to antenatal testing for HIV, but it
is important to remember that there may be a variety of reasons
for women's reluctance to be tested for HIV or to disclose their
HIV status or the factors which place them at risk of infection.
Fear of judgemental attitudes and actions by staff may be a factor inhibiting disclosure; also, some women may be unaware of
their exposure (Brierley 1993).

Table 6.2   Regional distribution of pregnancies in HIV infected
women reported since June 1989 (up to May 1994) (RCOG 1994)

Region	Total pregnancies
Thames regions	270
Rest of England, Wales and Northern Ireland	98
Scotland	243
Irish Republic	84
Total	695

The Department of Health has issued guidelines (DoH 1994) to encourage the more extensive testing for HIV in pregnancy in those areas where there is a high prevalence amongst the antenatal population. Voluntary named antenatal testing for HIV, it is argued, will allow women and their partners time to consider all the relevant options for care during and after pregnancy. Specialist medical referral can be organised for the woman with HIV infection and the options of prophylactic treatment for opportunist infections, antiretroviral therapy and possible interventions to reduce the risk of transmission to the baby can be discussed. In particular, advice to HIV positive women not to breastfeed can contribute to reducing perinatal transmission.

In areas of lower HIV infection prevalence, it is suggested that testing for HIV in pregnancy should be selective, on the basis of known possible exposure, related to activities such as IVDU or a sexual partner at high risk of infection.

This guidance offers a framework for the development of testing services; how this is implemented and to what extent it remains sensitive and responsive to the needs of pregnant women depends on the strategies adopted by the midwives implementing it.

□ Principles for antenatal testing for HIV

Any testing programme, whether it is aiming for comprehensive testing of the antenatal population or more selective provision of testing, must be guided by the same principles:

- Early provision of good, easily understood information to all women, preferably sent to them prior to their booking appointment, on the basis of which they can make a choice as to whether or not to have an HIV test;
- Sufficient provision of well informed staff with adequate time to offer an opportunity for discussion of testing with a woman before she decides;
- The ability to report results back to women at an identified time and adequate services for the post-test counselling and support of women who are identified as HIV positive;
- A well defined referral pattern for women who are found to be HIV positive so that their care, during pregnancy and subsequently, is well co-ordinated and maximises the benefits of early diagnosis.

The aim of a testing programme, as well as enabling diagnosis of HIV infection when that is sought by a woman, should be to educate women about HIV infection, how it is acquired and how transmission of HIV might be prevented. It is only on the basis of good information that a woman can make informed reproductive choices, including that of being tested for HIV, and decisions about activities which may place her at risk of HIV infection in future.

While there may be advantages to antenatal HIV testing, including early intervention and treatment of maternal opportunist infections, antiretroviral treatment if indicated, avoidance of breastfeeding and prophylactic treatment for the newborn, it must be remembered that the diagnosis of HIV, particularly during pregnancy, can have profoundly negative effects on a woman's social, emotional and psychological circumstances, and the importance of these cannot be overlooked (Brierley 1993).

■ The implications of HIV infection during pregnancy

Consideration of the implications of HIV for the health of the pregnant woman and her baby centres on a number of key issues:

- The effect of pregnancy on the course of HIV disease;
- The effect of HIV on the progress and outcome of pregnancy;
- The factors influencing transmission of HIV from mother to child (vertical transmission);
- Implications of HIV infection for the health of the baby.

On the basis of a growing understanding of the interaction between HIV infection and pregnancy and the factors influencing vertical transmission from mother to child, it is beginning to be possible to define objectives for care in pregnancy which might reduce the likelihood of transmission from mother to child.

□ The effect of pregnancy on the course of HIV disease

As noted in a previous contribution to this series (Roth & Brierley 1990), the extent to which pregnancy adversely alters the course of a woman's HIV infection remains undecided. As yet, few studies have compared the natural history of the infection in pregnant and non-pregnant women.

There is a theoretical concern that the interaction of HIV infection with pregnancy, which in itself alters immune function, might provoke acceleration of the infection (Schoenbaum *et al* 1988).

A number of prospective studies have failed to demonstrate marked advance of HIV illness during pregnancy in women with asymptomatic infection (MacCallum *et al* 1988; Schoenbaum *et al* 1988; Johnstone *et al* 1992) in spite of early impressions that this might have been the case. There may, however, be some evidence for an acceleration of immune compromise during pregnancy (Schaefer *et al* 1988). Further research charting the natural course of infection in women, both pregnant and not, is required (Minkoff & DeHovitz 1990; Berer 1993).

A recent study reported from Haiti (Deschamps *et al* 1993), monitored the health of 140 asymptomatic HIV seropositive women, over a mean period of 44 months. Forty-four of the women were pregnant or became pregnant as the study progressed and 96 were not pregnant. HIV-related signs and symptoms occurred in 68 per cent of the pregnant women and 35 per cent of the non-pregnant controls, with the mean time period until the appearance of the first HIV-related symptom similar in both groups although there was a trend toward earlier presentation of symptoms in the pregnant women. AIDS developed in 32 per cent of the pregnant women and 19 per cent of the controls. Twenty-seven per cent of the pregnant women and 15 per cent of the non-pregnant group died during the study period, all as a consequence of AIDS.

The study did not demonstrate any statistically significant differences between the two groups of seropositive women with regard to rates of progression to AIDS or death due to AIDS, but the researchers caution that the numbers were not large enough to provide conclusive information. Morbidity and mortality in both the pregnant and non-pregnant group was very high.

By including a non-pregnant control group, this study permitted comparison of the development of infection in pregnant and non-pregnant seropositive women. Significantly, the other methodological advantages which its authors identify – that it was not subject to 'confounding factors' such as IVDU, high rates of termination of pregnancy or the use of prophylactic medications – highlight the enormous variety of social, economic, health and political conditions in which HIV infection occurs, and the diversity of circumstances in which women are infected by and live with HIV. This has important implications for assessing the interrelationships between pregnancy and HIV and reinforces the need for caution regarding the extent to which findings in one context can be confidently extrapolated to another.

In her comprehensive review of this issue, Berer (1993)

advocates the adoption of global protocols to guide the design of research into HIV and pregnancy, noting the lack of comparability of existing studies because of the lack of standardisation in relation to maternal outcomes measured, period of follow-up and identification of co-factors. She notes the small size of many studies and the failure to control for age, parity, socioeconomic status, other risk factors for maternal mortality and morbidity, reproductive tract infections and injecting drug use, all of which might influence outcomes (Berer 1993: 18–19).

The evidence for acceleration of HIV-related disease in asymptomatic women is not strong. This may be different for the woman with AIDS. Women who become immune compromised as a consequence of HIV infection are vulnerable to serious, life-threatening infection during pregnancy (Minkoff *et al* 1990) and require close surveillance of immune status and prophylaxis or early treatment against opportunist infections as appropriate. Some retrospective studies identify a shorter survival time with AIDS in pregnant women, with the opportunist infection *pneumocystis carinii* pneumonia (PCP) a leading cause of pregnancy-related deaths (reviewed in Bardequez & Johnson 1994). However, Johnstone and colleagues (1992), in their retrospective review of the clinical condition of women with AIDS in Edinburgh, did not find differences in the clinical presentation, severity of illness or laboratory findings between pregnant and non-pregnant women. Further large scale prospective studies are required to clarify the effect of pregnancy on progression in symptomatic and asymptomatic HIV positive women.

A woman's decision about continuation and the progress of the pregnancy should be based on a full physical and immunological assessment and the opportunity to discuss her concerns with medical staff.

□ **The effect of HIV infection on pregnancy outcome**

With regard to the impact of HIV infection on pregnancy, there is no evidence of marked differences in the outcome of comparable pregnancies of asymptomatic HIV positive and HIV negative women in a number of studies in developed countries (Johnstone *et al* 1988, Selwyn *et al* 1989).

However, findings have been different in different circumstances. The perinatal outcome for a group of infants born to HIV-positive mothers in Zaire amongst whom the rate of AIDS was 18 per cent, was characterised by higher rates of prematurity, low birthweight and higher neonatal death rates than in a comparable group of babies born to HIV-negative mothers (Ryder *et al* 1989).

■ Transmission of maternal HIV infection to the fetus/newborn

Evidence of transmission of HIV from a mother to her fetus and newborn baby has been well documented, as is the variation of transmission rates in different populations (Newell & Peckham 1994).

The on-going multicentred European prospective study, which has reported on 831 infants born to HIV positive women in 19 European centres since the end of December 1984, currently estimates the rate of maternal to child transmission to be 14.4 per cent (European Collaborative Study 1992); other European studies suggest a rate of transmission up to 20 per cent (Newell & Peckham 1994). Transmission rates in Africa are estimated to be about 30 per cent, while the range for the USA is quoted as 16–30 per cent (Newell & Peckham 1993).

Such differences in reported transmission rate may be due in part to differences in study design; those which include children who were diagnosed after birth will bias the rate of transmission upwards. But, there is evidence suggesting that there are differences between populations in terms of risk factors of maternal transmission, such as the mother's clinical and immunological status during pregnancy, coexisting maternal infections, gestational age at delivery, mode of delivery, infant feeding, and other as yet unidentified factors (Newell & Peckham 1994).

□ The routes and timing of vertical transmission of HIV

While it is clear that vertical transmission may occur either during pregnancy, at the time of birth, or postnatally, sound evidence for the relative importance of each of these periods and the factors influencing transmission are only slowly emerging.

□ Transmission during pregnancy

HIV has been detected in fetal tissue as early as eight and twenty weeks of pregnancy (Jovaisas *et al* 1986; Lewis *et al* 1990). It has been isolated from cervical secretions (Vogt *et al* 1986), amniotic fluid and placental tissue at 15 weeks of pregnancy (Sprecher *et al* 1986) and cord blood at term (Ryder *et al* 1988), all of which provide evidence for transmission *in utero*.

☐ **Transmission during birth**

A number of recent studies have produced evidence suggesting that the intrapartum period may be of particular significance for vertical transmission of HIV (Ehrnst *et al* 1991; Goedert *et al* 1991; Krivine *et al* 1992).

Krivine and colleagues (1992), who conducted a prospective study of 50 infants of HIV-1 positive mothers, detected serological evidence of HIV infection in only five infants at birth, but by the age of 4–9 weeks, 16 infants were positive to HIV by polymerase chain reaction (PCR) and viral culture. These findings suggest active replication of HIV during the first weeks of life, supporting the hypothesis of transmission during late pregnancy or at delivery.

Demographic, clinical and epidemiological data on 66 sets of twins and triplets born to HIV infected women in nine different countries was retrospectively studied by Goedert *et al* (1991). Infection was more common in first-born than in second-born twins, both for those born by vaginal delivery and by caesarean section. The difference in infection rates between first and second twin was statistically significant in the case of vaginal delivery, suggesting that factors associated with proximity to and passage through the birth canal may contribute to the higher rate of infection in the first presenting twin.

A Swedish study (Ehrnst *et al* 1991) sought to investigate the relationship between maternal viraemia and vertical transmission of HIV. They found no convincing evidence of transmission of HIV in the first and second trimester of pregnancy. HIV was not isolated at birth from any of the 27 babies studied, but was identified in five of the babies by six months of age. They concluded that there is no consistent transmission of HIV across the placenta during maternal viraemia and that in most cases transmission occurs close to or at delivery.

The possibility also exists that transmission of HIV may occur at different times in different pregnancies, according to how advanced a woman's HIV infection is, with intrauterine transmission more common with more advanced maternal infection (Tibaldi *et al* 1993; Newell & Peckham 1993).

□ Transmission in the postnatal period

HIV has been detected in breast milk (Thiry *et al* 1985) and since 1985 a number of case reports have implicated breastfeeding as the source of HIV infection of infants born to mothers who were known to have become infected with HIV after delivery (Ryder & Hassig 1988).

Dunn *et al* (1992) have undertaken a systematic review of published studies which fulfilled criteria for determining the quantitative risk of transmission via breastfeeding. Analysis of the data from four studies of babies of mothers who acquired HIV infection after delivery, suggest that the risk of transmission from a postnatally infected breastfeeding woman to her child is 29 per cent.

Determination of the risk associated with breastfeeding for infants whose mothers were infected prenatally is more difficult, because of the impossibility of distinguishing between *in utero* or intrapartum transmission and postnatal transmission. However, from the data of five studies of infants of prenatally infected mothers, comparisons were made between rates of infection in breastfed and artificially fed infants. Calculations suggest that the additional risk of transmission by breastfeeding, over and above that of *in utero* or intrapartum transmission, is 14 per cent. The authors conclude that where safe alternatives to breastfeeding are available, HIV infected women should be discouraged from breastfeeding (Dunn *et al* 1992). However, in accordance with WHO/UNICEF guidance, where there are high rates of infant infection and high rates of malnutrition and infant mortality, breastfeeding should continue to be encouraged, regardless of the woman's HIV infection status (Global Program on AIDS 1992).

Van de Perre and colleagues (1993) investigated factors which might influence the transmission of HIV via breast milk. They enrolled 215 HIV-1 infected women at the time of delivery in Kigali, Rwanda. Milk was examined at 15 days, 6 months and 18 months postpartum for the presence of IgG, IgA and IgM, and for the presence of viral DNA in milk cells. Infection in the babies was defined according to serological and clinical criteria.

Those babies whose mothers did not have HIV-1 infected milk cells had a low risk of acquisition (18 per cent), similar to that of formula-fed babies; those babies fed on breast milk with infected cells, but no HIV-1 specific IgM had a high rate of HIV infection (47 per cent), while those babies fed on infected milk which also contained HIV-1 specific IgM had a rate of acquisition of 30 per cent (Van de Perre *et al* 1993).

The researchers anticipate that further research to test the hypothesis of the protective effect of IgM in breast milk could provide the basis for a strategy using vaccination to induce IgM immune response in women to reduce prenatal transmission.

☐ **Risk factors for transmission from mother to infant**

A study of 55 infants born to women in Brooklyn, New York (Goedert *et al* 1989) found a crude transmission rate to the neonate of 29 per cent, with infected babies much more likely to have been born before 38 weeks gestation. It remains to be established whether this association is a result of early *in utero* infection with HIV, perhaps predisposing to preterm delivery, or if prematurity increases the babies' risk of infection during the intrapartum and early postpartum period. While the study of Zairean women mentioned above (Ryder *et al* 1989) also found a higher rate of preterm delivery in the babies of HIV positive women, in the Brooklyn study the rate of preterm delivery amongst women who used IV drugs was similarly high in seropositive and seronegative women (Goedert *et al* 1989).

No association was found between infant infection and maternal T cell levels (CD4 and CD8), or anti-p24 levels, but there was a high reactivity to the virus envelope glycoprotein gp120 in those women who delivered babies at term and did not transmit the virus, a finding which may have importance for vaccine development and possibly for perinatal immunotherapy (Goedert *et al* 1989).

An analysis of risk factors for vertical transmission, based on 721 children born in 19 European centres, from the end of December 1984 to the beginning of August 1991 has been reported (European Collaborative Study 1992). The risk of infection was greatest among the infants born to 13 women with AIDS, but other HIV-related maternal illness was not predictive of transmission. Rates of transmission were higher for women with p24-antigenaemia and a CD4 count of less than 700 ml (European Collaborative Study 1992).

According to multivariate analysis, factors associated with increased risk of transmission included breastfeeding and birth before 34 weeks gestation. Vaginal deliveries in which scalp electrodes, forceps, or vacuum extractors were used were associated with higher transmission, but only in centres where such interventions were not routine. A lower transmission rate was associated with caesarean section, but there was insufficient detail regarding the circumstances of the intervention to draw any conclusions from this finding.

In subsequent analysis in the European Collaborative Study (1994) it has been estimated that caesarean section might halve the rate of HIV transmission. However, the authors point out the need to balance the potential protective effect of caesarean section against the risks and costs and the possibility that other strategies to reduce perinatal transmission, such as antiretroviral therapy and vaginal lavage, may prove to be effective and more attractive alternatives to caesarean section. They stress the need for the completion of randomised controlled trials to evaluate both mode of delivery and antiretroviral therapy to support the introduction of routine measures.

The French Prospective Multicentre Cohort study (Blanche *et al* 1994) examined the rate of disease progression in children with vertically acquired HIV infection and the stage of disease of the mother at the time of delivery. An infected child whose mother had AIDS was 3–4 times more likely to present with an AIDS indicator disease within the first 18 months of life compared with the children of asymptomatic mothers or those with persistent generalised lymphadenopathy.

□ Diagnosis and natural history of infection in infants

Whereas in adults the diagnosis of HIV infection can be achieved in most cases by detection of antibodies to HIV by means of an enzyme linked immunosorbant assay test (ELISA), confirmed by the Western Blot, in newborn infants diagnosis presents significant difficulties. All infants of HIV positive mothers will be born with passively-acquired antibodies to HIV; thus, regardless of the infant's own infection status, its HIV antibody test will be positive. Maternal antibodies may persist in the baby's circulation for up to 15–18 months, and therefore it is only after this time that a positive antibody test has diagnostic significance for the baby. In addition, it is difficult to culture HIV, a difficulty compounded in infants because of the limit to the size of a blood sample available for viral culture.

A number of techniques for the early detection of HIV have been devised, including the use of polymerase chain reaction (PCR), whereby viral DNA, if present, can be amplified to enhance detection (Rogers *et al* 1989), and the detection of HIV specific IgA antibodies in the infants blood (Weiblen *et al* 1990). However, no single test has yet been standardised or evaluated that can be relied on for the early diagnosis of all HIV infected infants (Brierley 1993).

Prospective study of children born to HIV infected women

Table 6.3 Signs and symptoms associated with HIV infection in babies born to HIV positive women (adapted from European Collaborative Study 1991)

- Oral candidiasis on two consecutive examinations at least two months apart
- A combination of two of these persisting for two months: lymphadenopathy, hepatomegaly, splenomegaly (LHS)
- Abnormal immunological findings:
  - Hyperimmunoglobinaemia
  - Low CD4/CD8 lymphocyte ratios

---

has contributed to a description of the natural history of HIV infection in infants, as well as analysis of the factors which are associated with transmission from mother to child (European Collaborative Study 1991; European Collaborative Study 1992; Nair *et al* 1993). Like so many features of HIV infection, findings vary depending on the maternal population studied.

In a prospective study of 134 infants born to HIV positive mothers in Baltimore, low birthweight, poor intrauterine growth, and neonatal infections were significantly more common in those babies found to be infected (Nair *et al* 1993). Maternal factors associated with HIV transmission to babies included a tendency to a higher rate of drug use during pregnancy, signs or symptoms of chorioamnionitis during labour, and a high prevalence of a variety of sexually transmitted diseases during pregnancy.

The European Collaborative Study (1991) reported results based on follow-up of 600 children born to HIV infected mothers in ten European centres up to June 1990. There were no differences in clinical features at birth between infected and uninfected children. However, amongst infected children followed up for 18 months or more, there was a tendency for those who acquired AIDS to have been born earlier, lighter and smaller for dates than those not developing AIDS, although these differences were not statistically significant.

The study found that oral candidiasis and parotitis occurred significantly more frequently in infected children; septicaemia and pneumonia with gram-negative bacteria were also strongly associated with HIV infection. There was a high incidence of abnormal immunological findings in children who went on to develop AIDS. On the basis of their findings it was concluded that, without a definitive virological diagnosis, it would be possible by monitoring of immunoglobins, CD4/CD8 ratio, and clinical signs to identify HIV infection in 48 per cent of infected children by 6 months of age, with a specificity of more than 99 per cent (European Collaborative Study 1991).

The emerging natural history of HIV infection suggests two patterns of disease progression in HIV infected children (Gibb & Wara 1994). During the first year of life, severe immunodeficiency associated with serious infections or encephalopathy occurs in 15–25 per cent of infected infants, while the remaining 75–85 per cent of infected infants have a more slowly progressive disease, similar to the adult pattern.

The uncertainty of diagnosis of the baby is a source of considerable extra stress to the families affected by HIV; continuity of care from midwives and doctors who are comfortable responding to their questions and expressions of anxiety is essential.

■ Monitoring and treatment of HIV infection during pregnancy

Surveillence of the woman's immune status during pregnancy is important, and CD4 and CD8 counts should be measured, at least in each trimester, in order to identify compromise of the immune system.

In asymptomatic women, when CD4 counts are less than $200/mm^3$, prophylactic treatment for *pneumocystis carinii* pneumonia (PCP), as well as the antiretroviral drug, zidovudine, are recommended (Kesson & Sorrell 1993). Therapy is available for opportunist infections associated with the immune compromise of HIV infection. Pathogens significant for pregnant women include Candida, cytomegalovirus (CMV), Mycobacterium tuberculosis, *pneumocystis carinii, toxoplasmosis gondii, cryptococcus neoformans* and *cryptosporidium*. Early recognition and treatment are essential if the benefits of intervention are to be optimised.

Clinical examination and history taking during antenatal visits might elicit evidence of opportunist infection or other signs of disease progression, such as fever, night sweats, weight loss or excessive fatigue. Attention should be paid to reports of dysphagia and sore mouth, and the mouth examined for signs of candidal infection and hairy oral leukoplakia. Regular examination for lymphadenopathy should be carried out. Dyspnoea, cough or tachypnoea may signal PCP which is frequently insidious in its onset. Intestinal infection may occur and present with abdominal pain, diarrhoea or vomiting.

Herpes simplex and herpes zoster infections are common and will require treatment. Other skin lesions may be present that require investigation and treatment.

In women whose immune status is compromised inquiry about

visual disturbances and retinal examination is important to exclude CMV or candidal infections of the retina.

Attention should be paid to signs of vaginal infection and investigation and treatment initiated, in order to reduce the risks associated with chorioamnionitis and preterm rupture of membranes.

☐ The use of zidovudine during pregnancy

Experience has been accumulating of the use of antiretroviral and other treatments for women with HIV disease during pregnancy. A number of studies have investigated the effects of zidovudine on the fetus and newborn.

Sperling and colleagues (1992) reviewed the pregnancies and outcomes of 43 women who had been given zidovudine during pregnancy. The retrospective review concluded that the drug was well tolerated by the pregnant women, 24 of whom had it for two trimesters of pregnancy. Use of the drug was not associated with malformations in the newborns, premature birth or fetal distress. No pattern of haematological abnormalities in the babies was detected, but the growth retardation and anaemia seen in a minority of babies may have been related to their mothers' treatment with zidovudine. This study included only a small number (12) of fetuses exposed during the first trimester, and cannot be used to predict the potential teratogenic risk (Newell & Peckham 1994).

Subsequently, a multiphase trial was initiated (O'Sullivan *et al* 1993), the first stage of which set out to study the safety and pharmokinetics of zidovudine in mothers and infants during parenteral and oral zidovudine administration to HIV-1 infected, asymptomatic women during the third trimester, labour and delivery. The pharmokinetics of the drug was similar in pregnant women to that in non-pregnant adults, while the drug had a half-life in the neonate ten times that in the mother. No significant adverse effects on the baby were noted at birth or during the 18 month follow-up period.

News of the preliminary results of a multicentred study focusing on the effect of zidovudine on perinatal transmission is reported in the Morbidity and Mortality Weekly Report (1994). The multicentred study (ACTG 076) randomly allocated HIV infected women, who were between 14 and 34 weeks' gestation, and who had no other indications for zidovudine treatment (i.e. their CD4+ lymphocyte counts were greater than 200 cells/mm^3), to receive either zidovudine (100 mg five times daily) during pregnancy and labour, or placebo, and their babies to receive the same treatment for the first six weeks of life. The trial was terminated when analysis of interim data demonstrated a two-thirds reduction in the perinatal transmission rate in the treatment group (Morbidity & Mortality Report 1994). In February 1994, the National Institutes of Health in the USA alerted doctors to the findings, stressing their direct applicability only to women sharing the characteristics of those in the study. The need to exclude any long term toxicity has been noted (Lancet Editorial 1994), and careful long term follow-up of the babies will be required to assess the long term efficacy and safety of this intervention.

□ General considerations for care

In its essential features, there is little to add to the principles of care for women with HIV infection outlined by Roth and Brierley (1990). Improved understanding of the natural history of HIV infection in mothers and babies, as well as a more refined understanding of the factors promoting transmission, will open possibilities for intervention that may protect maternal health during pregnancy and reduce infection in the baby.

The numbers of women whose pregnancies are complicated by HIV are bound to increase for the forseeable future; it is up to midwives to make good use of their involvement with the care of these women in order to improve the value of that care to them and their families and the women who follow them.

■ Recommendations for clinical practice in the light of currently available evidence

1. Sound information about HIV infection and the issues relevant to pregnancy should be provided to all women, in a language and form they can understand.
2. Women should have the opportunity to discuss HIV testing, its advantages and disadvantages, with well informed staff, and HIV testing should be available. Women should not have to identify themselves as 'at risk' in order to be given information.
3. The protection of confidentiality and privacy at the time of discussion, in relation to the documentation in notes and in all subsequent care, is essential.

4. Provision for the post-test counselling, support and specialist medical assessment and treatment of women who are known to be HIV positive or are diagnosed during pregnancy must be available. Access to community based support groups should be facilitated.
5. Women should be informed of the additional risk of transmission to the baby associated with breastfeeding.
6. Continuity of midwifery and obstetric care should be ensured thoughout pregnancy, delivery and postnatal care. Aims of care include early detection and treatment of intercurrent infection, early awareness of immune compromise and avoidance of invasive procedures during labour, as well as adequate support and information throughout pregnancy and the postnatal period.
7. Contact with a paediatrician should be established and discussion of follow-up and possible prophylactic treatment of the baby should take place before delivery.
8. Decisions about antiretroviral, prophylactic therapy and other interventions should be made by the woman in consultation with a specialist physician, on the basis of assessment of her immunological status, general health and currently available research evidence.

■ Practice check

- Does your unit provide adequate information for women, on the basis of which they can make informed choices about HIV testing? Is it in a form which they can understand and take time to consider?
- Is there adequate privacy and time available for women to comfortably discuss their concerns? Are there informed midwives or health advisors available?
- How is (or would) an HIV sample be sent and a diagnosis be recorded in order to protect the confidentiality of the woman? What measures are in place to prevent accidental disclosure?
- Are standards and procedures for universal precautions (Roth & Brierley 1990: 160–61) in dealing with potentially infectious body fluids followed in your practice? What would be required to achieve this?
- Are you familiar with local and national support for HIV positive women and is that information made readily available to women?

• Is your unit able to provide women with care which is not judgemental and which is sensitive to their complex needs?

□ **Acknowledgements**

This chapter would be incomplete without reference to my good friend and collaborator, Janette Brierley, with whom this chapter was intended to be written.

Janette, who died tragically in November 1993, was a continuing source of inspiration to colleagues and clients on a wide range of midwifery issues. She made a particular contribution by seeking to identify and focus on the women-centred concerns thrown up by HIV infection and encouraging midwives to respond to the professional challenges posed by HIV infection, always keeping the interests and needs of women very clearly in view.

■ References

Ades AE, Davison CF, Holland FJ, Gibb DM, Hudson CN, Nichols A, Goldberg D, Peckham CS 1993 Vertically transmitted HIV infection in the British Isles. British Medical Journal   306: 1296–9

Bardequez A, Johnson MA 1994 Women and HIV-1 infection. AIDS   8 (suppl 1): S261–73

Berer M 1993 Women and HIV/AIDS. An international resource book. Pandora, London

Brierley J 1993 HIV and AIDS in childbirth: are midwives responding to the needs of women? Midwives Chronicle   106 (1268): 317–25

Blanche S, Mayaux MJ, Rouzioux C *et al* 1994 Relation of the course of HIV infection in children to the severity of the disease to their mothers at delivery. New England Journal of Medicine   330: 308–12

Chin J 1990 Current and future dimensions of the HIV/AIDS pandemic in women and children. Lancet   336: 221–4

Concorde Coordinating Committee 1994 Concorde: MRC/ANRS randomised double-blind controlled trial of immediate and deferred zydovudine in symptom-free HIV infection. Lancet   343: 871–81

Department of Health 1994 Guidelines for offering voluntary named HIV antibody testing to women receiving antenatal care. HMSO, London

Deschamps MM, Pape JW, Desvarieux M *et al* 1993 A prospective study of HIV-seropositive asymptomatic women of childbearing age in a developing country. Journal of Acquired Immune Deficiency Syndromes   6(5): 446–51

Dunn DT, Newell ML, Ades AE, Peckham CS 1992 Risk of human immunodeficiency virus type 1 transmission through breastfeeding. Lancet 340: 585–8

Ehrnst A, Lindgren S, Dictor M *et al* 1991 HIV in pregnant women & their offspring: evidence for late transmission. Lancet 338: 203–7

European Collaborative Study 1991 Children born to women with HIV-1 infection: natural history and risk of transmission. Lancet 337: 253–60

European Collaborative Study 1992 Risk factors for mother-to-child transmission of HIV-1. Lancet 339: 1007–12

European Collaborative Study 1994 Caesarean section and the risk of vertical transmission of HIV-1 infection. Lancet 343: 1464–7

Expert Maternity Group 1993 Changing childbirth. HMSO, London

Gibb D, Wara D 1994 Paediatric HIV infection. AIDS 8 (suppl 1): S275–83

Global Program on AIDS 1992 Current and future dimensions of the HIV/AIDS pandemic: a capsule summary. WHO, Geneva

Goedert JJ, Mendez H, Drummond JE *et al* 1989 Mother-to-infant transmission of human immunodeficiency virus type 1: association with prematurity or low anti-gp 120. Lancet ii: 1351–4

Goedert JJ, Duliege AM, Amos CI *et al* 1991 High risk of HIV-1 infection for first born twins. Lancet 338: 1471–5

Hankins CA 1990 Issues involving women, children and AIDS primarily in the developed world. Journal of Acquired Immune Deficiency Syndromes 3: 443–8

House of Commons Health Committee 1992 Second report: Maternity Services Vol. 1. HMSO, London

Johnstone FD, MacCallum L, Brettle R *et al* 1988 Does infection with HIV affect the outcome of pregnancy? British Medical Journal 296: 467

Johnstone FD, Willox L, Brettle RP 1992 Survival time after AIDS in pregnancy. British Journal of Obstetrics and Gynaecology 99: 633–6

Jovaisas E, Koch MA, Schafer A 1986 LAV/HTLV-III in a 20 week fetus (letter). Lancet ii: 1129

Kesson A, Sorrell T 1993 Human immunodeficiency virus infection in pregnancy. Baillière's Clinics in Obstetrics & Gynaecology 7(1): 45–74

Krivine A, Ghislaine F, Linsen C *et al* 1992 HIV replication during the first weeks of life. Lancet 339: 1187–9

Lancet Editorial 1994 Zidovudine for mother, fetus, and child: hope or poison? Lancet 334 (8917): 207–9

Lewis SH, Reynolds-Kohler C, Fox HE *et al* 1990 HIV-1 in trophoblastic and villous Hofbauer cells and haemotological precursors in eight-week fetuses. Lancet 335: 565–8

Lipsky JJ 1994 Commentary: Concorde lands. Lancet 343: 866–7

MacCallum LR, France AJ, Jones ME, Steel CM, Burns SM, Brettle RP *et al* 1988 The effects of pregnancy on the progression of HIV infection. IV International Conference an AIDS. Stockholm, June 1988; abstract 4032

Minkoff HL, De Hovitz JA 1990 Care of women infected with the human immunodeficiency virus. Journal of the American Medical Association 261(9): 1289–94

Minkoff HL, Willoughby A, Mendez H *et al* 1990 Serious infections during pregnancy among women with advanced immunodeficiency virus infection. American Journal of Obstetrics and Gynecology 162(1): 30–4

Morbidity and Mortality Weekly Report 1994 Zidovudine for the prevention of HIV transmission from mother to infant. Morbidity and Mortality Weekly Report 43: 285–7

Nair P, Alger L, Hines S *et al* 1993 Maternal and neonatal characteristics associated with HIV infection in infants of seropositive women. Journal of Acquired Immune Deficiency Syndromes 6: 298–302

Newell ML, Peckham C 1993 Risk factors for vertical transmission of HIV-1 and early markers of HIV-1 infection in children. AIDS 7: S591–7

Newell ML, Peckham C 1994 Working towards a European strategy for intervention to reduce vertical transmission of HIV. British Journal of Obstetrics and Gynaecology 101: 192–6

O'Sullivan MJ, Boyer PJJ, Scott GB *et al* 1993 The pharmokinetics and safety of zidovudine in the third trimester of pregnancy for women infected with human imunodeficiency virus and their infants: Phase I Acquired Immunodeficiency Syndrome Clinical Trials Group study (protocol 082). American Journal of Obstetrics and Gynecology 168: 1510–16

Pratt R 1991 AIDS: a strategy for nursing care 3rd edn. Edward Arnold, London

Public Health Laboratory Service 1993 Unlinked anonymous monitoring of HIV prevalence in England and Wales: 1990–92. Communicable Disease Report Review 3(1): 8

Rogers MF, Thomas PF, Starcher ET *et al* 1987 Acquired immunodeficiency syndrome in children: Reports of the Centers for Disease Control national surveillance, 1982–1985. Pediatrics 79: 1008–14

Rogers MF, Chin-Yih O, Rayfield M *et al* 1989 Use of the polymerase chain reaction for early detection of the proviral sequences of human immunodeficiency virus in infants born to seropositive mothers. New England Journal of Medicine 320: 1649–54

Roth C, Brierley J 1990 HIV infection – a midwifery perspective. In Alexander J, Levy V, Roch S (eds) Intrapartum care: a research-based approach (Midwifery Practice Vol 2). Macmillan, Basingstoke

Royal College of Obstetricians and Gynaecologists 1994 National study of HIV in pregnancy. Newsletter 20, September 1994. RCOG, London

Ryder RW, Hassig S 1988 The epidemiology of perinatal transmission of HIV. AIDS 2 (suppl 1): S83–9

Ryder RW, Nsa W, Behets F, Vercauteren G, Baende E *et al* 1988
Perinatal transmission in two African hospitals: one year follow-up.
IV International Conference on AIDS, Stockholm, June 1988,
abstract 4128

Ryder RW, Nsa W, Hassig S *et al* 1989 Perinatal transmission of
the human immunodeficiency virus type 1 to infants of
seropositive women in Zaire. New England Journal of
Medicine 320: 1637–42

Schaefer A, Grosch-Woener I, Friedmann W, Kunze R, Mielke M,
Jiminez E 1988 The effects of pregnancy on the natural course of
the HIV infection. IV International Conference on AIDS,
Stockholm, June 1988, abstract 4039

Scharf E 1992 Research: HIV, AIDS and the invisibility of women. In
O'Sullivan S, Thomson K (eds) Positively women. Sheba, London

Schoenbaum EE, Davenny K, Selwyn PA 1988 The impact of
pregnancy on HIV-related disease. In Hudson C, Sharp F (eds)
AIDS and obstetrics and gynaecology. Proceedings of the 19th
Royal College of Obstetricians and Gynaecologists Study Group.
RCOG, London

Selwyn PA, Schoenbaum EE, Davenny K, Robertson VJ, Feingold AF
et al 1989 Prospective study of human immunodeficiency virus
infection and pregnancy outcomes in intravenous drug users.
Journal of the American Medical Association 261(9): 1289–94

Sperling RS, Stratton P, O'Sullivan MJ *et al* 1992 A survey of
zidovudine use in pregnant women with human immunodeficiency
virus infection. New England Journal of Medicine 326: 857–61

Sprecher S, Soumenkoff G, Puissant F *et al* 1986 Vertical
transmission of HIV in 15-week fetus. Lancet 2: 288–9

Thiry L, Sprecher-Goldberger S, Jockheer T *et al* 1985 Isolation of
AIDS virus from cell free breast milk of three healthy virus
carriers. Lancet ii: 891–2

Van de Perre P, Simonon A, Hitimana D *et al* 1993 Infective and
anti-infective properties in breastmilk from HIV-I-infected women.
Lancet 341: 914–18

Vogt MV, Witt DJ, Craven DE *et al* 1986 Isolation of HTLVIII/LAV
from cervical secretions of women at risk for AIDS. Lancet
1: 525–7

Weiblen BJ, Lee FK, Cooper ER *et al* 1990 Early diagnosis of HIV
infection in infants by detection of IgA HIV antibodies.
Lancet 335: 988–90

■ Suggested further Reading

Berer M, Ray S 1993 Women and HIV/AIDS. An international
resource book. Pandora, London

Brierley J 1993 HIV and AIDS in childbirth: are midwives

responding to the needs of women? Midwives Chronicle   106: 317–25

Bury J, Morrison V, McLachlan S 1992 Working with women and AIDS: medical, social and counselling issues. Routledge, London

O'Sullivan S, Thomson K (eds) 1992 Positively women. Sheba, London

Positively Women 1994 Women Like us: Positively Women's Survey on the needs and experiences of HIV positive women. Positively Women, London

Pratt R 1991 AIDS: a strategy for nursing care 3rd edn. Edward Arnold, London

Roth C, Brierley J. 1990 HIV infection – a midwifery perspective. In Alexander J, Levy V, Roch S (eds) Intrapartum care: a research-based approach (Midwifery Practice Vol 2). Macmillan, Basingstoke

Chapter 7

Postnatal perineal care revisited

Jennifer Sleep

Following delivery, the activity and excitement which accompany the moment of birth are often superseded by a time of quiet enchantment. For many parents, the experience of labour is momentarily forgotten as they delight in the miracle of their newborn. These are precious moments for the new family, moments to be savoured and treasured. This is a time when the midwife should safeguard the couple's privacy, if only for a brief span, before reality intervenes.

The postnatal period is a time when each mother has to adjust to physical changes and new emotional demands. These two aspects are inextricably linked; a woman cannot tenderly cuddle her baby whilst experiencing severe perineal pain, neither can she feel herself to be an attractive desirable partner if she is incontinent of urine. Whilst acknowledging the interdependence of physical and psychological factors, this chapter largely seeks to explore the physical problems commonly reported by new mothers by reflecting on current practices in perineal care. Since first being published (Sleep 1990) this chapter has been revised and expanded to take account of recently published research evidence and to reflect changes in current practices in perineal care.

■ It is assumed that you are already aware of the following:

- The physiology of wound healing;
- The anatomy of the pelvic floor;
- Which drugs are secreted in breast milk.

132

■ Perineal pain in the early postnatal period

Perineal pain in the early days following childbirth is one of the most common causes of maternal morbidity. There is evidence to suggest that 23 per cent of women report some degree of discomfort 10 days following normal delivery (Sleep *et al* 1984). This discomfort and pain is not solely confined to mothers who sustain perineal trauma. In this large randomised trial Sleep and colleagues found pain to be equally reported by two groups of women despite a 10 per cent increased intact perinea rate in one of these groups. It is, therefore, important to recognise that perineal pain is a source of distress and discomfort whatever the mode of delivery or the extent of perineal trauma and this may severely jeopardise the woman's recovery and adversely affect the relationship with her partner for a considerable period of time. The problem, therefore, has consequences for tens of thousands of women every year in Britain alone.

During this ten day period, the midwife maybe the only health professional to be in daily contact with the mother either in hospital or at home. Mothers are therefore most likely to turn to their midwife for advice about the best way to alleviate this distressing problem. This leads to direct or indirect prescribing by midwives. Direct prescribing includes specific treatments such as bath additives or herbal preparations which are available through many retail outlets; indirect prescribing requires medical sanction for pharmaceutical products including some analgesics and electrical therapies but the request is often instigated by the midwife.

□ Oral analgesics

There is a confusing choice of pharmacological preparations which can be taken by mouth to relieve pain. Several factors need to be considered in selecting the most appropriate agent.

1. The severity of pain to be treated
It is helpful to use a simple categorical or visual analogue scale which can be easily used by mothers to assess their pain. For example, a categorical scale may allow the pain to be rated as mild, moderate or severe. Kremer and colleagues (1981) suggest that such scales are reliable and valid but tend to lack sensitivity. An alternative method is a 10 centimetre visual analogue scale which offers a wider spectrum of responses which may be more sensitive to the woman's experience of pain. However, the

same authors suggest that as many as 7 per cent of the the population would not be able to cope with the demand of completing such a scale. It is, therefore, important to bear this in mind
in terms of appropriateness of use – for example, for women
who do not speak English as a first language or those who have
limited understanding. A numerical rating scale or pain ther-
mometer offers a useful alternative (Downie *et al* 1978). Postpartum
perineal pain is usually reported by women to be mild or moderate when classified on one of the above scales, although a small
number of mothers report the experience as severe. The choice
of analgesia should thus offer flexibility of prescribing to provide appropriate and adequate relief of pain in each of these
categories.

2.   The extent to which the drug is secreted in breast milk
If the drug is secreted in breast milk, consideration should also
be given to whether this holds any potential danger for the baby.

3.   The risk of side-effects
The risks of maternal side-effects, such as gastric upset or constipation, need to be considered.

4.   Cost
Midwives should be aware of the relative costs of alternative preparations. There is anecdotal evidence to suggest a wide variation
in what midwives advise for perineal pain. In a survey of 50 English
maternity units (Sleep & Grant 1988a), midwives reported that
their first line management was usually oral analgesia (78 per
cent). There was a clear consensus that paracetamol was the
analgesic of choice for mild to moderate pain (96 per cent).
This seems a sensible option for nursing mothers as the drug is
largely free of unwanted side-effects. (Drugs & Therapeutics
Bulletin 1986). A stock is available in most maternity units and
it can be bought over the counter at many shops. A useful alternative may be one of the nonsteroidal, anti-inflammatory agents
such as ibuprofen (largely retailed under the brand name of
Brufen); little is secreted in breast milk and this too may now
be bought across the counter, marketed as Nurofen or Cuprofen.
The main disadvantage of these drugs is the cost (500 × 200 mg
Brufen tablets could be bought for approximately £3.52 in 1994
while 500 × 500 mg paracetamol tablets were nearer £1.80 in
price at the same time). In this survey there was, however, no
agreement about which oral analgesic should be given for more
severe pain (see Table 7.1). The most popular choices were combinations of paracetamol or aspirin with another analgesic, most

Table 7.1 Oral analgesics for perineal pain

	Consultant units N = 36 (%)	GP units N = 14 (%)	All units N = 50 (%)
Mild/moderate pain			
paracetamol	35 (97)	13 (93)	48 (96)
More severe pain			
co-proxamol (Distalgesic) – paracetamol 325mg + dextropropoxyphene 32.5mg	7 (19)	2 (14)	9 (18)
co-dydramol (Paramol) paracetamol 500mg + dihydrocodeine 10mg	5 (14)	1 (1)	6 (12)
co-codaprin (Codis) – aspirin 400 mg + codeine phosphate 8mg	4 (11)	2 (14)	6 (12)
co-codamol (Paracodol; Panadeine) – paracetamol 500mg + codeine phosphate 8mg	1 (3)	2 (14)	3 (6)
dihydrocodeine tartrate 30mg (DF 118)	2 (6)	0 (0)	2 (4)
papaveretum (Omnopon) + aspirin	2 (6)	0 (0)	2 (4)
mefanamic acid 250mg (Ponstan)	2 (6)	0 (0)	2 (4)
buprenorphine 0.2mg (Temgesic)	1 (3)	0 (0)	1 (2)
ibuprofen 200mg (Brufen)	1 (3)	0 (0)	1 (2)

commonly a codeine derivative. Given its tendency to cause constipation, codeine does not seem the ideal choice in this circumstance especially when other effective alternatives are available. In a replicative survey conducted in one large district hospital Harris (1992) found that co-dydramol (a codeine compound) was still in widespread use for the relief of severe pain. One useful alternative codeine-free analgesic is dextropropoxyphene which, in combination with paracetamol, is marketed as Distalgesic although it is less popular than it used to be because of the risk of dependence and overdose. These risks would appear minimal in relation to the efficacy of the preparation in relieving perineal pain especially when the more potent analgesic is likely to be required for a relatively short period of time. The combination of an opioid such as papaveretum (Omnopon) with aspirin may be particularly useful for more severe pain. Although concern is widely expressed regarding the potential risk in exposing the baby to aspirin via the mother's milk, the drug is secreted only in low concentrations (Briggs *et al* 1986) so it may be worth considering its occasional use as a means of improving maternal comfort.

■ **Cleanliness and hygiene**

Vulval swabbing and bathing are widely recommended, both as prophylactic measures in reducing the risks of infection and for the relief of perineal discomfort.

In a survey of mothers who were questioned on their tenth day following delivery, 93 per cent (1674 women) reported that bathing had relieved their discomfort (Sleep & Grant 1988b). This observation was uncontrolled, however, so it is not known whether a similar proportion of women would have gained relief if they had not bathed at all or used showers rather than baths. This may be an important issue especially when many maternity units are supplied with bidets, and showers are increasingly fitted in modern units and many new homes.

A survey of womens' experiences and midwives' practices conducted on behalf of the National Childbirth Trust (Greenshields & Hulme 1993) reported that 24 per cent of mothers (191) considered that one or more combination of these various modes of cleaning had effectively reduced their discomfort. So clearly, for some women, using a bath or shower does prove to be therapeutic. There does, however, appear to be little consensus in the advice given to mothers by midwives regarding the frequency of perineal cleaning although, for the most part, the mothers themselves are probably well able to decide their own schedule.

Only one randomised trial (Ramler & Roberts 1986) has reported a comparison between warm and cold sitz baths. Cold sitz baths were more effective in relieving discomfort especially immediately following the birth. In practice, however, it is difficult to imagine that many women would willingly choose cold, rather than warm, water as a therapeutic soak. Indeed 119 of the 159 women approached to enter the trial refused to participate in this study; the main reason given was their (understandable) reluctance to immerse themselves in cold water.

One of the oldest 'remedies' for perineal and other trauma is the addition of salt to the bath water. Sleep and colleagues (1984) reported that as many as 33 per cent of women were adding salt to their bath water ten days after normal delivery. Salt is believed to soothe discomfort and to speed the healing process, but its precise mode of action is unclear. Claims that it has antibacterial or antiseptic properties remain unsubstantiated (Ayliffe *et al* 1975). There is little consensus as to the amount of salt to be used; recommended quantities range from a heaped tablespoon in a small bath (Marks & Ribeiro 1983) to 3 lbs in 3 gallons of water (Houghton 1940). In the only published trial (Sleep & Grant 1988b), 1800 women were randomly allocated to one of three bathing policies; 600 mothers were asked to add measured quantities of salt to the bath water, 600 were asked to add a 25 ml sachet of Savlon bath concentrate and the remaining group were asked not to add anything to their baths in the ten days following delivery.

Overall, 89 per cent of the the women complied. There was little, if any difference between the three groups in terms of perineal pain or relief afforded at either ten days or three months postpartum. The patterns of wound healing were also similar in the three groups. On the basis of these results there is no case for recommending the use of salt or Savlon bath additive as a means of reducing maternal discomfort following delivery. An additional factor to be taken into account is the cost of these preparations; 100 women using additives once a day for 10 days would spend £80 on Savlon or about £8 on salt.

One recently published randomised controlled trial compared the use of two preparations of lavender oil with an inert oil added to the bathwater following childbirth (Dale & Cornwell 1994). No statistical or clinical difference was reported by the mothers in terms of reduced perineal discomfort within the first ten days postpartum.

The use of hairdriers in the drying of the perineum after washing is another widely recommended practice. There is little consensus as to whether the hairdrier should blow hot or cold air. Some advocate its use with conviction, whilst others raise serious doubts about its usefulness, or indeed its harmlessness (Wheeler 1988). There is at least a theoretical possibility that the drying effect applied to the sensitive, moist skin of the perineum may have a harmful effect which may result in increased pain and possibly delayed healing. There is no evidence that this is the case: on the other hand there is no evidence that this practice is safe. This procedure is in need of urgent evaluation.

□ Local applications

Midwives possess an armoury of topical remedies used for the symptomatic relief of perineal pain. Many of these are recommended on a trial and error basis and are met with varying degrees of success; few have been subjected to formal evaluation.

In 1988, Sleep and Grant (1988a) reported icepacks as the most commonly used local treatment (84 per cent of units). This evidence was supported in the NCT survey (Greenshields & Hulme 1993). These packs are usually made from frozen water filled fingers of rubber gloves, crushed ice or alternatively, a packet of frozen peas may be used which offers the added advantage of moulding to the body contours. Ice packs do appear to give symptomatic relief by numbing the tissues but this effect usually lasts for a very short period of time and there is no clear evidence of any long term benefit. Indeed the accompanying vasoconstriction may delay wound healing. There are also concerns that, as solid icepacks are difficult to position accurately at an anatomical site such as the perineum (especially in postnatal women who are for the most part ambulant), 'ice burns' may occur as a result of contact with the skin and surrounding tissues. For these reasons it may be preferable to use crushed ice 'sandwiched' between layers of a pad which may then be applied for restricted periods of time when the mother is able to rest.

□ Anaesthetics

These are currently available in a range of base carriers including aerosol sprays, gels, cream or foam. The agent of choice appears to be lignocaine. Three randomised trials have been reported assessing a variety of spray formulae each containing lignocaine. In the first of these (Harrison & Brennan 1987a), alcoholic aerosol formulations of 5 per cent lignocaine and 2 per cent cinchocaine were compared with water only placebo spray in a single dose study in 76 primiparae. Both anaesthetics were clearly more effective than water in relieving discomfort. Of the two active preparations lignocaine was marginally more efficient. In the second trial (Harrison & Brennan 1987b), lignocaine was used in both an aqueous and an alcoholic base; the aqueous preparation appeared slightly more effective than the alcoholic sprays containing either lignocaine or cinchocaine. The results of the third study confirm this finding (Harrison & Brennan 1987c). The analgesic effectiveness of 5 per cent aqueous lignocaine spray was superior to the alcoholic formulation and comparable to a single 500 mg dose of mefanamic acid (Ponstan). The only reported side-effect was transitory stinging following application of the alcoholic spray which may prove a deterrent to their repeated use by women following childbirth. Lignocaine in a gel form has also been compared with an inactive aqueous cream (BNF) applied in the first 48 hours after delivery. The mothers who applied lignocaine reported less pain and better pain relief (Hutchins *et al* 1985). There are claims that the repeated application of local anaesthetics in close proximity to mucous membranes can cause irritation and local sensitisation leading to discomfort. No evidence can be found to substantiate these claims. In the absence of such evidence it would seem that lignocaine, in an aqueous base, could prove a useful application for women in the relief of perineal discomfort. The gel formulation has the added advantage of being considerably cheaper – and ozone friendly. Prices for 1994 suggest that lignocaine spray would be four times more expensive than 2 per cent lignocaine gel containing 0.25 per cent chlorhexidine.

□ **Combinations of local anaesthetics and topical steroids**

It can be assumed that local oedema and inflammation are major contributory factors to perineal pain. In recent years pharmaceutical preparations have been developed and introduced into clinical care amidst enthusiastic claims for their efficacy in reducing these problems. Epifoam (Stafford Miller Ltd) is one such vigorously marketed product; it contains pramoxine hydro-chloride 1 per cent and hydrocortisone acetate 1 per cent in a water-miscible muco-adhesive foam base. The only encouraging results on the use of this preparation have been from studies which were uncontrolled (Nenno & Loehfelm 1973; Bouis *et al* 1981) or unsatisfactorily controlled (Goldstein *et al* 1977). In the only well controlled, double-blind study published to date (Greer & Cameron 1984) mothers in the Epifoam group reported more oedema and a greater use of oral analgesia, particularly after the third day, than mothers in the control group who used a simple aqueous foam. Wound breakdown was also more common in the actively treated group. In this study, outcome was assessed by an observer who did not know the trial allocation thus minimising assessor bias.

Steroids are known to impair wound healing (Walter & Israel 1979) so it is biologically plausible that Epifoam may cause longer term problems in relation to perineal healing. Furthermore, it is costly (£3 per 12 gm cannister was the approximate

1994 price), and Hutchins and his colleagues (1985) did not feel that the very marginal effectiveness over lignocaine suggested by their study warranted the extra expense. In the light of present evidence, it is questionable whether this product does have the benefits claimed for it; it should therefore not be recommended or prescribed for mothers until subjected to further longer term evaluation in properly controlled trials (Drugs and Therapeutic Bulletin 1987).

☐ **Herbal remedies**

An ever increasing number of herbal preparations aimed at relieving perineal discomfort is currently available through many retail outlets. Their growing popularity probably reflects a belief that 'natural' remedies must be safe. Some are produced in tablet form, others are recommended for infusion and external application. There is however a dearth of evidence to support their efficacy or safety (Ehudin-Pagano *et al* 1987).

Arnica (leopard's bane) is supplied as tablets. As it is claimed to stimulate tissue repair and to reduce bruising following childbirth a course of treatment is recommended to begin at the onset of labour or as soon after delivery as possible (Ford 1988). A small unpublished pilot study using a double-blind experimental design suggests that in the short term, arnica may be of limited value (Holwell 1993).

Chamomile and comfrey are both believed to aid healing; the latter may be steeped to form a solution which can then be mixed with slippery elm and applied to the perineum as a paste or added to bath water as a soothing soak (Bunce 1987). Swabbing of the perineum with tincture of calendula (marigold) is also recommended because it is believed to have antiseptic properties, hence its advocated use also on the cord stump of the neonate. Rare cases of hypersensitivity to calendula have been reported (Drugs & Therapeutics Bulletin 1986).

In a Survey conducted by Sleep and Grant (1988a), 12 per cent of units reported the use of pads soaked in witch hazel as a locally applied compress. Two randomised trials have assessed this practice. Spellacy (1965) randomly allocated mothers to use either pads soaked in witch hazel and glycerine solution or pads soaked in tap water. The majority of women in each group reported some symptomatic relief but there was no evidence that the witch hazel/glycerine combination proved any more effective in relieving perineal discomfort than plain tap water. The second trial (Moore & James 1989) was conducted in Bristol during

1986. Three hundred women who had forceps deliveries were randomly allocated to one of three treatment groups; witch hazel, icepacks and Epifoam. There was some evidence that witch hazel was the most effective analgesic on the first day of use, but by day three icepacks were the most satisfactory. Thereafter there were no clear differences between the treatment groups up to the final six weeks assessment. However, as this study was poorly controlled and incompletely reported, the results must be interpreted with caution.

Some herbal remedies may be potentially useful in helping mothers to recover after childbirth, however their widespread use needs to be approached with the same caution as the introduction of pharmaceutical products. Evidence is required that they are safe and therapeutic – both in the short term in relieving pain and in the longer term in not compromising or delaying healing.

□ Electrical therapies

Ultrasound and, to a lesser extent, pulsed electromagnetic therapy are being used increasingly in the first few days after delivery to relieve perineal pain and discomfort. In a telephone survey of 36 consultant units and 14 GP units (Sleep & Grant 1988b), 36 per cent of units reported using ultrasound, 12 per cent used heat and 6 per cent used pulsed electromagnetic energy. These therapies were more frequently available at consultant rather than GP units.

The mechanisms by which therapeutic ultrasound may improve tissue repair and reduce pain have been reviewed by Dyson (1987). The precise mode of action is not properly understood but there is evidence that it is effective for some soft tissue injuries, such as tennis elbow (Binder *et al* 1985), leg ulcers (McDiarmid *et al* 1985; Callam *et al* 1987) and following oral surgery (El Hag *et al* 1985). Two small trials assessing its use for perineal trauma (McLaren 1984; Creates 1987) have been incompletely reported. The transducer head is applied directly to the skin and must be moved gently throughout the transmission to minimise tissue damage by heating and air cavitation; conduction is aided by the use of a couplant jelly or cream. The therapy requires constant operator attendance and so is costly in physiotherapists' time.

Pulsed electromagnetic energy is also claimed to improve wound healing and reduce pain. One of the greatest practical advantages of the treatment lies in its ease of application. It may be transmitted through a sanitary towel, so obviating the need for bedside attendance, although for safety's sake the physiotherapist needs to remain in the vicinity whilst any electrical treatment is in progress. One published study evaluating its use in perineal care suggests that active therapy accelerates the resolution of bruising (Bewley 1986). In this trial 100 mothers were randomly allocated to receive a treatment from one of two machines, one active and the other inactive. By day three of the trial, however, the author comments that it became obvious to the operators which was the 'active' machine. This may therefore have introduced observer bias on the part of the physiotherapists as well as influencing the mothers' expectations of the therapy. Perineal pain reported by the mothers before and after completion of treatment failed to reveal any benefit from the active therapy.

Both of these electrical therapies were evaluated in a trial where each mode of treatment was compared in a 'double-blind' design (Grant *et al* 1989). Four hundred and fourteen women with moderate or severe perineal trauma were randomly allocated to receive active ultrasound, active pulsed electromagnetic energy, or corresponding placebo therapies. Operator, subject and assessor bias were minimised by using a twelve point dial on each machine: eight settings were active, four were inactive. The codes for the switches were held in sealed envelopes and changed at two monthly intervals to minimise risk of participants breaking the operating code; the output of the machines was tested weekly by someone who worked in a different part of the hospital. Therapy was started within 24 hours of delivery, a maximum of three treatments being given during a 36 hour period. Mothers assessed their pain before and after each treatment, at ten days and at three months postpartum. Overall, more than 90 per cent thought that treatment made their problem better. Bruising looked more extensive following ultrasound therapy but then seemed to resolve more quickly but mothers did not report less pain as a consequence. More pain was reported by mothers who had received pulsed electromagnetic energy therapy at ten days postpartum (see Table 7.2), although by three months following delivery there were no reported differences in outcome. Neither treatment had an effect on perineal oedema or haemorrhoids. In the light of these results current enthusiasm for these new therapies should be tempered. Further controlled trials are needed to replicate this design and to assess different machine settings and length of treatment.

Table 7.2 Ultrasound and pulsed electromagnetic therapies for perineal trauma: outcome 10 days after delivery

	Pulsed electro-magnetic energy (N = 129)		Ultrasound (N = 134)		Placebo (N = 131)	
	N	(%)	N	(%)	N	(%)
Perineal pain in last 24 hours*						
(reported by mother)						
None	33	(26)	53	(40)	48	(37)
Mild	57	(44)	50	(37)	44	(34)
Moderate	30	(23)	24	(18)	33	(25)
Severe	9	(7)	7	(5)	6	(5)
Use of pain-killers in previous 24 hrs	31	(24)	30	(22)	25	(19)
Community midwife's assessment						
Perineal wound breaking down	6	(5)	6	(4)	3	(2)
Haemorrhoids	33	(26)	35	(26)	33	(25)
Bruising	22	(17)	14	(10)	18	(14)
Oedema	13	(10)	10	(7)	11	(8)

*$P < 0.05$

☐ The use of cushions and rings

The use of rubber or sorbo rings continues to be favoured by both midwives and mother alike. There appears to be no sound evidence to support the commonly held belief that that these comfort aids impede circulation and pre-dispose mothers to the risks of thrombosis (Church & Lyne 1994), but neither is there confirmatory evidence that they may be used safely during the postnatal period. One recently marketed pressure relieving cushion the Valley cushion (U.T. Care Products Ltd), offers the potential advantages of combining pressure relief with minimal compression of blood vessels. This is achieved by the V shape of the cushion so that the buttocks are supported in the arms of the V allowing the perineum to be relieved of direct pressure. To date, however, the product has not been formally evaluated.

□ Pelvic floor exercises

The main reason for teaching and encouraging women to perform pelvic floor muscle exercise is to prevent urinary stress incontinence and genital prolapse. It has been argued that pregnancy and childbirth may be precipitating or aggravating factors for stress incontinence. Certainly the symptom is a source of considerable embarrassment and distress to women. The most marked difference is between nulliparous and parous women; 60 per cent of primiparae experience the symptom for the first time during pregnancy (Stanton *et al* 1980); for multiparae there seems to be relatively little increase in severity until parity reaches four or more (Thomas *et al* 1980). In a large scale survey of 11 701 women, MacArthur and colleagues (1991) reported that 1782 women (15.2 per cent) recorded the first onset of stress incontinence within three months immediately following delivery. Urinary frequency was reported by a further 5.7 per cent of mothers. Few of these bladder problems were transient; 75 per cent reported that the symptom persisted a year later. Clearly, the problem is a major source of morbidity for mothers, yet in this same study only 14 per cent of women had sought medical advice for these symptoms. It would seem, therefore, that the midwife has an important role to play in:

- Reducing the 'at risk' factors associated with stress incontinence, for example a first stage of labour lasting longer than ten hours or second stage longer than two hours (MacArthur *et al* 1991);
- Raising women's awareness of this potential problem;
- Encouraging mothers to seek advice at an early stage and not to suffer the problem as a 'natural consequence' of childbirth.

In a midwifery study of 1000 mothers following normal, vaginal deliveries, 19 per cent reported some degree of involuntary loss of urine three months postpartum (Sleep *et al* 1984). Two contentious issues arise in relation to urinary incontinence and childbirth; perineal trauma at delivery as a precipitating or aggravating factor, and the role of pelvic floor exercises as both a preventative and a curative therapy.

There is a growing body of evidence to suggest that the risk of incontinence is not directly related to the extent of trauma to the perineal tissues at delivery (Yarnell *et al* 1982; Gordon & Logue 1985). A longer term follow-up of 1000 women, conducted three years following normal deliveries (Sleep & Grant 1987),

Table 7.3 Urinary incontinence three years after participation in a randomised trial of restrictive versus liberal use of episiotomy

	Restrictive policy N = 329 (%)		Liberal policy N = 345 (%)	
Involuntary loss of urine				
Less than once a week	69	(22)	82	(25)
1–2 times in last week	37	(12)	35	(11)
3 or more times in last week	6	(2)	7	(2)
Sufficiently severe to wear a pad				
– sometimes	26	(8)	24	(7)
– everyday	5	(2)	4	(1)
Loss of urine when coughing, laughing or sneezing	103	(33)	105	(31)
Loss of urine when urgent desire to pass urine but no toilet nearby	41	(13)	41	(13)

did not provide evidence to support the hypothesis that the liberal use of episiotomy prevents urinary incontinence (see Table 7.3). Several authors have suggested that the faecal and urinary incontinence result from damage to the innervation of pelvic floor muscles, rather than stretching *per se* (Snooks *et al* 1984; Swash 1988). Whatever the underlying cause, weakness of the pelvic floor muscles, as judged by an inability to contract them voluntarily and effectively, often accompanies stress incontinence (Shepherd 1983). Exercises aimed at increasing awareness and improving tone are therefore often recommended and taught both during pregnancy and following childbirth. There is some evidence that the more successfully the exercises are performed, the better the results (Shepherd 1983). It is, however, difficult to know whether the muscles are being contracted effectively without inserting a finger into the vagina or the use of a teaching aid such as a perineometer gauge. The latter consists of a rubber device resembling a foley catheter or a condom which can be inserted into the vagina and inflated until the woman is just conscious of pressure. As the levator muscles are contracted, so the squeeze pressure registers in cm water on the gauge thus enabling the woman to know whether or not she is contracting the muscles effectively.

Neither of these strategies would seem to be appropriate for women in the early weeks following delivery when the vagina and surrounding tissues may be bruised and sore for some considerable time.

Few formal attempts have been made to evaluate the role of pelvic floor exercises in this context. One such study, however, was conducted in 1985 (Sleep & Grant 1987). The aim of this study was to compare the postnatal exercise programme currently in operation in the West Berkshire Health District with a scheme which reinforced this initial instruction during the immediate postpartum period. The reinforcement programme comprised additional teaching sessions, positive encouragement by community midwives and health visitors, and attempts to enhance motivation by personal contact and the use of an exercise diary for one month. The main hypothesis was that the more intensive programme would reduce the incidence of urinary incontinence three months after delivery. Assessment also included the effect of the programme on perineal discomfort and the mothers' reported feelings of general wellbeing. One thousand, eight hundred women entered the trial and were randomly allocated to one of the two policies. By the time of the community midwife's visit on the tenth postnatal day, mothers in the intensive group were more likely to have performed their exercises than mothers allocated to the normal policy (78 per cent versus 68 per cent). This difference was greater three months after delivery (58 per cent versus 42 per cent). At three months postpartum, one in five women admitted some degree of urinary incontinence (5 per cent needing to wear a pad for some or all of the time), and 3 per cent had faecal incontinence. These frequencies were very similar in the two groups allocated different exercise policies. One of the differences observed was in the perineal pain reported three months following delivery. This was not, however, reflected in differences in dyspareunia or in the timing of resumption of sexual intercourse (see Table 7.4). The results of this study, therefore, do not support the primary hypothesis, and this in turn raises questions about the value and content of the exercise programmes currently offered to women around the time of childbirth. Gordon and Logue (1985) suggest that regular physical exercise which women find both interesting and fun (for example, swimming, dancing or keep fit programmes) might prove more therapeutic in the long term than encouraging them to practice specific pelvic floor exercises. It is possible that the substantial resources involved in teaching the current pre- and postpartum programmes could be used more effectively. Even a relatively small reduction in the incidence of this distressing condition is potentially important. Further well designed studies are therefore needed to assess alternative strategies aimed at prevention and treatment.

Table 7.4 Perineal symptoms at three months postpartum

	Normal exercises N = 793 (%)		Intensive exercises N = 816 (%)	
Pain in the past week**	101	(12.7)	76	(9.3)
– mild	69	(8.7)	60	(7.4)
– moderate	28	(3.5)	15	(1.8)
– severe	4	(0.5)	1	(0.1)
Time to resumption of sexual intercourse				
– in first month	263	(33.2)	249	(30.5)
– in second month	351	(44.3)	380	(46.6)
– in third month	67	(8.4)	85	(10.4)
– too painful	13	(1.6)	9	(1.1)
– not attempted	90	(11.3)	85	(10.4)
– not recorded	9	(1.1)	8	(1.0)
Intercourse painful at first	368	(46.4)	391	(47.9)
Intercourse still painful	154	(19.4)	167	(20.5)

** X_2 (1df) for trend = 7.14; $p < 0.01$

■ Faecal incontinence and control of flatus

Within the past decade there has been an increasing awareness of the problem of faecal incontinence arising as a consequence of childbirth. In a large trial, Sleep and Grant (1987) reported a prevalence of 3 per cent, three months post partum. The precise aetiology is as yet, poorly understood but clearly, midwives need to be aware of this potential problem. The NCT survey (Greenshields & Hulme 1993) highlights that, for many women, controlling flatus after delivery may represent a distressing problem. Over one quarter of the respondents (500 mothers) reported this to be a difficulty, although the majority (80 per cent) also reported that the symptom had been present during the antenatal period. Nevertheless, it is important that midwives are aware of this source of distress and are able to reassure mothers that the effects are likely to be transient.

■ Haemorrhoids and constipation

Haemorrhoids frequently occur during pregnancy and following delivery. In their survey, MacArthur and colleagues (1991) reported an overall prevalence of the problem in 18 per cent of women following childbirth, 8 per cent of whom reported the occurrence for the first time within three months of delivery. Only 16 per cent of the 931 cases had subsided within three months; 70 per cent of these women reported that the symptoms had lasted for more than a year whilst 67 per cent described haemorrhoids as a problem up to nine years later. The midwife clearly has an important role to play both in the prevention and early treatment of this extremely painful and debilitating condition in order to reduce the risk that this will become a chronic problem. In one of the few reported studies to use haemorrhoid size as an outcome measure of treatment, two of the most commonly used electrical therapies, (namely ultrasound and pulsed electromagnetic energy), did not provide any relief for women in the early days following childbirth (Grant *et al* 1989); their use would thus appear not to be beneficial.

It is difficult to consider haemorrhoids in isolation from constipation following delivery as each will exacerbate the other if one of the problems is left untreated. Both conditions are clearly best prevented if at all possible. Previous reference has already been made to the importance of avoiding analgesics containing codeine; nutritional advice regarding a high fibre diet with fresh fruit supplements should also be encouraged, and the postnatal prescribing of oral iron preparations carefully reviewed.

■ Recommendations for clinical practice in the light of currently available evidence

1. There is little evidence to support many of the midwifery practices or the advice mothers receive relating to perineal care following childbirth. Overall, the quality of personal, individualised postpartum care is likely to be a major influence in reducing perineal pain and speeding recovery.
2. The use of a postnatal pain rating scale, to be completed by the mother, would provide an important tool for measuring the effectiveness of analgesia.
3. Paracetamol would currently appear to be the analgesic of choice. If this proves ineffective, a nonsteroidal anti-inflammatory agent such as ibuprofen may prove a useful

alternative. For more severe pain, drugs containing a
codeine derivative should be avoided and combined agents
such as oral papaveretum and aspirin considered.

4. Mothers appear to find bathing both therapeutic and
   desirable. If an ardent preference is expressed for the use
   of an additive such as salt, there is no evidence that this
   will prove harmful. As its addition does not appear to
   confer any specific benefit, however, its use need not be
   advocated.

5. The local application of ice should be approached with
   caution. Cooling with crushed ice should be considered for
   short periods only, preferably applied while the mother is
   resting. Tap water and witch hazel may be useful
   alternative cooling agents. The application of a local
   anaesthetic such as 5 per cent lignocaine spray or
   lignocaine gel are also effective in reducing discomfort and
   may last longer. The addition of a steroid to such topical
   preparations should be avoided as this may impair healing
   considerably in the long term.

6. The use of herbal remedies should also be approached
   with caution. On the whole there is no good evidence that
   they are beneficial and some may prove to be harmful.

7. On the basis of evidence currently available personalised
   physiotherapy services such as therapeutic ultrasound,
   pulsed electromagnetic energy and the teaching of pelvic
   floor exercises may prove beneficial largely as a
   consequence of the sympathetic, individualised support
   offered rather than the therapies themselves.

8. Preventative measures to minimise the risks of both
   constipation and haemorrhoids should be instigated as
   soon as possible following delivery.

9. Overall what emerges is the need for midwives to give, and
   for mothers to receive, kindness, respect, understanding,
   and patience. This is especially important in the early days
   following childbirth. Such a supportive environment should
   not be created as an 'optional extra available to some
   women because of their special needs . . . but one which is
   an integral part of the organisational framework of the
   service' (Ball 1987). Such concepts of care then become
   'woman centred', rather than routine or treatment centred,
   and may have a substantial impact in minimising pain and
   discomfort and promoting physical recovery and self-
   confidence. This is the midwifery challenge.

■ **Practice check**

- What oral analgesics are most commonly prescribed for nursing mothers on your unit? What is the rationale for this choice? When was the policy last reviewed?
- In your health district have the midwives defined and documented standards of care relating to aspects of postnatal perineal management?
- Is an audit tool currently being used to measure the achievement of standards of care offered by the midwives on your unit community base? How could such a tool be used to promote good practice?
- Is there a way in which you and your colleagues can use some of the available sound research evidence related to perineal care as a means of achieving Target 9 as highlighted in 'A vision for the future' document (DoH 1993): 'By the end of the year providers should be able to demonstrate at least three areas where clinical practice has changed as a result of research findings'.

☐ **Acknowledgement**

The author gratefully acknowledges the support of colleagues at the National Perinatal Epidemiology Unit, Oxford, in particular Dr Adrian Grant, Epidemiologist, without whose help much of this work would not have been undertaken.

■ **References**

Ayliffe GAB, Babb JR, Collins RJ, Davies J, Deverill C, Varney J 1975 Disinfection of baths and bathwater. Nursing Times 71(37) supplement: 22–3

Ball JA 1987 Reactions to motherhood. Cambridge University Press, Cambridge

Bewley EL 1986 The megapulse trial at Bristol. Association of Chartered Physiotherapists in Obstetrics and Gynaecology Journal 58:16

Binder A, Hodge G, Greenwood AM, Hazleman BL, Page P, Thomas DP 1985 Is therapeutic ultrasound effective in treating soft tissue lesions? British Medical Journal 290: 512–14

Bouis PJJ, Martinez LA, Hambrick TL 1981 Epifoam (hydrocortisone acetate) in the treatment of post episiotomy patients. Current Therapeutic Research 30: 912–16

Briggs GG, Freeman RK, Yaffe SJ 1986 Drugs in pregnancy and lactation. Williams & Wilkins, London

Bunce KL 1987 The use of herbs in midwifery. Journal of Nurse–Midwifery 32: 255–9

Callam MJ, Harper DR, Dale JJ, Ruckley CV, Prescott RJ 1987 A controlled trial of weekly ultrasound therapy in chronic leg ulceration. Lancet ii: 204–6

Church S, Lyne P 1994 Research-based practice: Some problems illustrated by the discussion of evidence concerning the use of a pressure-relieving device in nursing and midwifery. Journal of Advanced Nursing 19: 513–18

Creates V 1987 A study of ultrasound treatment to the painful perineum after childbirth. Physiotherapy 73: 162–5

Dale A, Cornwell S 1994 The role of lavender oil relieving perineal discomfort following childbirth: a blind randomised clinical trial. Journal of Advanced Nursing 19: 89–96

Department of Health 1993 A vision for the future. The nursing, midwifery & health visiting contribution to health and health care. NHSME, London

Downie WW, Leatham PA, Rind VM, Wright V, Branco JA, Anderson JA 1978 Studies with pain rating scales. Annals of Rheumatic Diseases 37: 378–81

Drugs and Therapeutics Bulletin 1986 Herbal medicines – safe and effective? Drugs and Therapeutics Bulletin 24: 97–100

Drugs and Therapeutics Bulletin 1987 Epifoam after childbirth for perineal pain. Drugs and Therapeutics Bulletin 25:39–40

Dyson M 1987 Mechanisms involved in therapeutic ultrasound. Physiotherapy 73: 116–20

Ehudin-Pagano E, Paluzzi PA, Ivory LC, McCartney M 1987 The use of herbs in nurse-midwifery practice. Journal of Nurse–Midwifery 32. 260–2

El Hag M, Coghlan K, Christmas P, Harvey W, Harris M 1985 The anti-inflammatory effects of dexamethazone and therapeutic ultrasound in oral surgery. British Journal of Oral Maxillofacial Surgery 23: 17–23

Ford J 1988 Postnatal homeopathic treatment. Midwives Chronicle 101(1206): 222–4

Grant A, Sleep J, McIntosh J, Ashurst H 1989 Ultrasound and pulsed electromagnetic energy treatment of perineal trauma: a randomised placebo-controlled trial. British Journal of Obstetrics and Gynaecology 96: 434–9

Greenshields W, Hulme H 1993 The perineum in childbirth – a survey of women's experiences and midwives' practices. National Childbirth Trust, London

Greer IA, Cameron AD 1984 Topical pramoxine and hydrocortisone foam versus placebo in relief of postpartum episiotomy symptoms and wound healing. Scottish Medical Journal 29: 104–6

Gordon H, Logue M 1985 Perineal muscle function after childbirth. Lancet ii 123–35

Goldstein PJ, Lippmann M, Leubehusen J 1977 A controlled trial of two local agents in postepisiotomy pain and discomfort. Southern Medical Journal 70: 806–8

Grant A, Sleep J, McInstosh J, Ashurst H 1989 Ultrasound and pulsed electromagnetic energy treatment for perineal trauma: a randomised placebo-controlled trial. British Journal of Obstetrics and Gynaecology 96: 434–9

Harris M 1992 The impact of research findings on current practice in relieving post partum perineal pain in a large district general hospital. Midwifery 8: 125–31

Harrison RF, Brennan M 1987a Evaluation of two local anaesthetic sprays for the relief of post-episiotomy pain. Current Medical Research Opinion 10: 364–9

Harrison RF, Brennan M 1987b A comparison of alcoholic and aqueous formulation of local anaesthetic as a spray for the relief of post-episiotomy pain. Current Medical Research Opinion 10: 370–74

Harrison RF, Brennan M 1987c Comparisons of two formulation of lignocaine spray with mefanamic acid in the relief of post-episiotomy pain: a placebo-controlled study. Current Medical Research Opinion 10: 375–9

Holwell D 1993 An evaluation of arnica for perineal pain after childbirth. Unpublished MSc dissertation, University of Surrey, Guildford

Houghton M 1940 Aids to practical nursing. Baillière Tindall & Cox, London

Hutchins CJ, Ferreira CJ, Norman-Taylor JQ 1985 A comparison of local agents in the relief of discomfort after episiotomy. Journal of Obstetrics and Gynecology 6: 45–56

Kremer E, Atkinson JH, Ignelzi RJ 1981 Measurement of pain: patient preference does not confound pain measurement. Pain 10: 241–8

Marks J, Ribeiro D 1983 Silicone foam dressings. Nursing Times 79(19): 58–60

MacArthur C, Lewis M, Knox EG 1991 Health after childbirth. HMSO, London

McDiarmid T, Burns PN, Lewith GT, Machin D 1985 Ultrasound and the treatment of pressure sores. Physiotherapy 71: 66–70

McLaren J 1984 Randomised controlled trial of ultrasound therapy for the damaged perineum. Clinical Physics and Physiological Measurement 5:40

Moore W, James DR 1989 A random trial of three topical analgesic agents in the treatment of episiotomy pain following instrumental delivery. Journal of Obstetrics and Gynecology 10: 35–9

Nenno DJ, Loehfelm G 1973 Clinical trial of a topical foam for episiotomies. Medical Times 101: 123–5

Ramler D, Roberts J 1986 A comparison of cold and warm sitz baths for relief of postpartum perineal pain. Journal of Obstetric, Gynecologic and Neonatal Nursing 15: 471–4

Shepherd AM 1983 Management of urinary incontinence: prevention or cure? Physiotherapy 69: 109–10

Sleep J, Grant A, Garcia J, Elbourne D, Spencer JAD, Chalmers I 1984 West Berkshire perineal management trial. British Medical Journal 289: 587–90

Sleep J, Grant A 1987 Pelvic floor exercises in post-natal care – the report of a randomised controlled trial to compare an intensive exercise regimen with the programme in current use. Midwifery 3: 158–64

Sleep J, Grant A 1988a The relief of perineal pain following childbirth: a survey of midwifery practice. Midwifery 4: 118–22

Sleep J, Grant A 1988b Routine addition of salt or savlon bath concentrate during bathing in the immediate postpartum period – a randomised controlled trial. Nursing Times 84(21): 55–7

Snooks SJ, Setchell M, Swash MM, Henry MM 1984 Injury to innervation of pelvic floor musculature in childbirth. Lancet ii: 546–50

Spellacy W 1965 A double blind control study of a medicated pad for relief of episiotomy pain. American Journal of Obstetrics and Gynecology 92: 272

Stanton SL, Kerr-Wilson R, Grant Harris V 1980 The incidence of urological symptoms in normal pregnancy. British Journal of Obstetrics and Gynaecology 87: 897–900

Swash M 1988 Childbirth and incontinence. Midwifery 4: 13–18

Thomas MT, Plymat KR, Blanin J, Meade TW 1980 Prevalence of urinary incontinence. British Medical Journal 281: 1243–5

Wheeler K 1988 Perineal wound healing (letter). Midwives Chronicle 101(1200): 14

Yarnell JWG, Voyle JG, Sweetnam PM, Milbank J, Richards CJ, Stephenson TP 1982 Factors associated with urinary incontinence in women. Journal of Epidemiology and Community Health 36: 58–63

■ **Suggested further reading**

Grant A, Sleep J 1989 Relief of perineal pain and discomfort after childbirth. In Chalmers I, Enkin M, Kierse MJNC (eds) Effective care in pregnancy and childbirth: 1347–59. Oxford University Press, Oxford

Kitson A 1994 Post-operative pain management: a literature review. Journal of Clinical Nursing 3: 7–18

Chapter 8

Hypoglycaemia in the neonate

Susan L. Smith

Prior to delivery the fetus is completely dependent upon the constant transfer of glucose across the placenta. Under normal circumstances when sufficient maternal glucose is available, this placental transport system meets all of the fetal glucose requirements; indeed, studies have shown that no significant glucose production can be demonstrated in the human fetus at term (Kalthan *et al* 1979). However if fetal demands cannot be met, for example in cases of maternal hypoglycaemia or placental insufficiency, then the fetus is capable of adapting both by using alternative energy fuels, such as ketone bodies, and also by initiating fetal hepatic glucose production (Bozzetti *et al* 1988).

At delivery, the placental supply of glucose is interrupted and the blood glucose level decreases. The newborn infant must then maintain glucose homeostasis by ensuring a balance between hepatic glucose output and peripheral glucose utilisation. If this delicate equilibrium is not achieved then disturbances of glucose homeostasis occur. These are recognised clinically by the presence of hypoglycaemia or hyperglycaemia. This chapter will present some of the current relevant research focusing on hypoglycaemia in order to enable the midwife to make informed decisions regarding effective and appropriate care and management and will also review the following areas: fetal and neonatal glucose metabolism; definition of hypoglycaemia; causes of hypoglycaemia; antenatal management and parentcraft teaching; prompt identification and recognition of those infants at risk; screening methods and diagnosis; strategies of treatment; and the long term sequelae and outcome following hypoglycaemia.

For the reader's reference, a glossary of terms is given in Figure 8.1.

154

■ **It is assumed that you are already aware of the following:**

- The regulation of blood glucose concentrations in the adult;
- Pathways of glucose metabolism.

■ **Fetal and neonatal glucose metabolism**

Glucose and lactate are the major carbohydrates which, along with amino acids serve as substrates for fetal metabolism and growth. Glucose crosses the placenta from maternal serum by facilitated diffusion prior to being taken up by the umbilical circulation. The fetus is completely dependent upon this constant transfer of glucose to meet its requirements and studies have shown that in normal circumstances no significant glucose production can be demonstrated in the human fetus at term (Kalthan *et al* 1979). Fetal concentrations of glucose vary directly with maternal concentrations production. However, the enzymes for gluconeogenesis are present in the fetus as early as the third month of gestation. If fetal energy demands cannot be met then the fetus is capable of adapting both by using alternative substrates, for example ketone bodies and by 'turning on' its endogenous glucose production. A recent study which examined the relationship between maternal and fetal glucose concentrations at mid gestation in humans suggested that fetal glucose production was induced by maternal hypoglycaemia (Bozzetti *et al* 1988).

Glycogen is the major form of stored carbohydrate in the fetus and, although glycogen synthesis begins as early as the ninth week of gestation, most glycogen is accumulated in the last seven

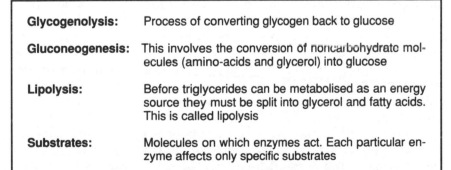

Glycogenolysis:	Process of converting glycogen back to glucose
Gluconeogenesis:	This involves the conversion of noncarbohydrate molecules (amino-acids and glycerol) into glucose
Lipolysis:	Before triglycerides can be metabolised as an energy source they must be split into glycerol and fatty acids. This is called lipolysis
Substrates:	Molecules on which enzymes act. Each particular enzyme affects only specific substrates

Figure 8.1 Glossary of terms

weeks of pregnancy and is synthesised from glucose. The major sites of glycogen deposition are liver, lung, heart and skeletal muscle. The rate of hepatic glycogen deposition varies with different species, depending on the period of gestation. In the human infant both skeletal muscle and hepatic stores reach three to five times adult levels by the end of gestation. They form, therefore, an important energy storage pool for the fetus and newborn infant. However, levels of glycogen in the lung and cardiac muscle decline as the fetus approaches term. This decrease in lung glycogen stores may reflect the energy requirement of ongoing developmental processes such as surfactant synthesis. Cardiac glycogen stores may serve as a significant energy source during periods of stress, for example survival after birth asphyxia does appear to be related to cardiac glycogen content (Mott 1961).

In addition to glycogen, the fetus also stores energy as adipose tissue. It is during the third trimester that most triglyceride synthesis takes place and, by full term, the fetus has a fat content of about 16 per cent. However, if the fetal glucose supply is decreased there will be a concomitant fall in the accumulation of adipose tissue.

Insulin is present in the pancreas of the human fetus by eight to ten weeks gestation. Because insulin does not cross the placenta, the increasing levels noted during the third trimester must reflect increased fetal pancreatic release (Hay 1991). Fetal insulin concentration does affect fetal glucose metabolism but it is probably more important as a growth factor. The fetuses of diabetic mothers have an increased pancreatic islet cell response to hypoglycaemia, releasing more insulin at any given blood glucose concentration. These higher insulin levels lead to increased growth, producing the macrosomia typically seen in infants of poorly controlled diabetic mothers. The related pancreatic hormone glucagon, which also does not cross the placenta, is present by the beginning of the second trimester. The role of glucagon in regulating fetal glucose metabolism is unclear and at normal fetal and maternal glucose concentrations, it does not appear to have a significant regulatory function. Although the actual concentration of glucagon in fetal blood is low, the high insulin:glucagon ratio may be important in preferentially maintaining glycogen synthesis and inhibiting gluconeogenesis, since glucagon is a potent inducer of gluconeogenic enzymes (Marsac 1976).

The role of lactate in fetal metabolism is relatively unclear. The finding of significant lactate concentrations in fetal blood was originally interpreted as a metabolic response to low fetal oxygen content. However, it is now recognised that lactate is synthesised in the placenta from other molecules – probably glucose from the maternal or fetal circulation and then taken up by the umbilical circulation.

At delivery a number of events take place which allow the neonate to assume its own glucose homeostasis. There are changes in circulatory insulin and glucagon levels as well as changes in their related receptors. These changes are accompanied by increases in enzyme activities essential for glycogenolysis and gluconeogenesis. Both serum glucagon and catecholamines increase threefold to fivefold, probably in response to cooling and cord cutting (Padbury *et al* 1981) and there is then a reversal of the fetal insulin:glucagon ratio. The elevated epinephrine and glucagon levels activate hepatic glycogen phosphorylase which induces glycogenolysis; simultaneously the decrease in glucose concentration stimulates hepatic glucose 6-phosphatase activity, which leads to an increase in hepatic glucose release. Increased catecholamines also stimulate lipolysis, providing substrate for gluconeogenesis. After a transient decrease immediately following birth, serum glucose levels rise, hepatic glycogen stores deplete and plasma fatty acid concentrations increase (reflecting lipolysis). Glucose homeostasis in the neonate also requires appropriate enzyme maturation and response.

The neonatal liver, in contrast to that of the fetus, is characterised by an increase in glycogen phosphorylase activity and a decrease in glycogen synthetase activity, consistent with rapid depletion of hepatic glycogen seen during the newborn period. Phosphoenolypyruvate carboxykinase (PEPCK) which is considered the rate-limiting enzyme required for gluconeogenesis also increases. This is probably a response to the reversal of the insulin:glucagon ratio, such that the glucagon concentration is greater than the insulin concentration (Girard 1986). Gluconeogenesis provides about 10 per cent of the glucose metabolised in the newborn in the few hours following birth (Frazier *et al* 1981). Thus, hormonal, receptor and enzyme activities in the fetus provide for anabolism and substrate accumulation, while those in the neonatal period provide for the maintenance of glucose homeostasis in response to the abrupt interruption of maternal glucose supply. The maintenance of glucose homeostasis depends on the balance between hepatic glucose output and peripheral glucose utilisation. Hepatic glucose output is a function of the rates of glycogenolysis and gluconeogenesis while peripheral glucose utilisation depends on the individual metabolic needs and demands placed on the neonate. If the rates of glycogenolysis and gluconeogenesis are not the same, either because of failure of the hormonal control mechanism or inadequacy of substrate supply, then disturbances of glucose homeostasis occur.

To summarise, the fetus relies on glucose supplied by the maternal circulation and lactate synthesised by the placenta to meet its metabolic needs and requirements for carbohydrate. At birth, the neonate must then provide carbohydrate to meet its glucose requirements by means of glycogenolysis and gluconeogenesis.

■ Definition of hypoglycaemia

There can be little doubt that the clinical problem of defining neonatal hypoglycaemia remains controversial (Koh *et al* 1988a). There have been various definitions since the first report from Europe in the early 20th century (Cobliner 1911). Reports in English began to appear in the early 1920s (Sedgwick & Ziegler 1920; Spence 1921). However, the results of these studies, which involved both full term and preterm infants, have since been considered 'normal' (Cornblath *et al* 1990). Later definitions in the 1960s were almost certainly influenced by feeding policies since it was then common practice for newborn infants not to receive feeds within the first day of life (Brown & Wallis 1963; Neligan *et al* 1963; Cornblath *et al* 1965). Although there was no clear definition for hypoglycaemia it was generally accepted that a symptomatic infant with a blood glucose concentration of 0–1mmol/l had an increased risk of brain damage (Haworth & McRae 1965).

The other significant issues at that time were firstly that the concept of infants being classified as 'small for gestational age' (SGA) had not been established and secondly that there were not defined policies for correcting hypoglycaemia using intravenous dextrose. In more recent years it has been recognised that with modern obstetric and neonatal care there have been changing patterns of 'normal blood glucose levels' (Srinivasan *et al* 1986; Hawdon *et al* 1992). Both these studies showed that, by three hours of age, full term infants had higher mean glucose levels than similar infants studied 25 years earlier and their results suggest that the definition of hypoglycaemia be revised upward accordingly. The controversy regarding the diagnosis continues with disagreement between senior medical staff (Cornblath *et al* 1990). In an attempt to establish the degree of variation, a study was undertaken in the late 1980s (Koh *et al* 1988a). In this particular study paediatric textbooks and the views of neonatologists were consulted. The study reviewed 36 paediatric textbooks and found that the definitions of hypoglycaemia ranged from 1.0–4.0mmol/l

(18–72 mg/dl) glucose. A total of 178 British paediatricians were asked their definition of hypoglycaemia. The majority used levels > 2 mmol/l (36 mg/dl) in full term infants and < 1.1 mmol/l (< 20mg/dl) in preterm or SGA infants. There is, however, no dispute among clinicians of the need to maintain blood glucose concentrations levels above a 'critical' level both in asymptomatic and symptomatic infants. Indeed, it has now been recognised that infants may well have abnormal clinical signs despite having glucose concentrations within the 'normal' range (Srinivasan *et al* 1986). It would seem more appropriate therefore, that for any given infant, hypoglycaemia should be defined as the blood glucose concentration at which the central nervous system glucose delivery falls below the cerebral glucose requirement.

However guidelines and recommendations (although pragmatic to some extent) remain important in the management of all infants. The most recent definition of hypoglycaemia of a glucose level of < 2.6 mmol/L (< 47 mg/dl), (Koh *et al* 1988b; Roberton 1992) is now generally accepted and used in clinical practice. However, this must be combined with clinical observation and experience in order to make an accurate and prompt diagnosis. Indeed, in the study mentioned by Koh *et al* (1988b) a small number of term infants demonstrated neurological dysfunction when blood glucose concentrations fell < 2.6 mmol/l irrespective of whether the infant was symptomatic, and, perhaps of even more significance is the fact that even when normoglycaemia was achieved, normal neurological function was not restored immediately.

■ Causes of hypoglycaemia

Most symptoms of hypoglycaemia are non-specific and could be attributed to other causes. It is important therefore that the midwife has the ability and knowledge to make an initial differential diagnosis. However, in some cases the actual diagnosis of hypoglycaemia will only become apparent when there is a resolution of symptoms following the administration of glucose. The differential diagnosis of neonatal hypoglycaemia can be divided into two groups – one where there is increased utilisation of glucose and the other where there is decreased hepatic production of glucose. In some cases there is a combination of the two. The chapter will look firstly at the causes of transient hypoglycaemia, including both decreased production of glucose and increased disappearance of glucose due to transient hyperinsulinism, and secondly will examine the causes of persistent or recurrent hypoglycaemia either due to increased utilisation or decreased production.

☐ Transient hypoglycaemia – decreased glucose production

Idiopathic The majority of cases of neonatal hypoglycaemia (95 per cent) fall in the category of asymptomatic transient hypoglycaemia which is frequently seen prior to the onset of feeding (Lilien *et al* 1991). It may therefore represent the normal decrease in glucose caused by the withdrawal of substrate supplied by the mother. It is the midwife's responsibility to ensure that newborn infants are able to maintain blood glucose concentrations and, in most cases, the baby will be ready to feed within the first hour after birth (Widstrom *et al* 1987). Recent studies have indicated that for healthy term infants during the first three postnatal days the prevalence of hypoglycaemia (blood glucose concentrations < 2.6 mmol/l) is 18 per cent (Hawdon *et al* 1992). However, healthy mature infants are not a major concern as they are able to respond to the hypoglycaemia by increasing hepatic glucose production and generating alternative fuels, such as ketone bodies. This response is under hormonal control, with suppression of insulin secretion and increased secretion of the counter-regulatory hormones – glucagon, cortisol and catecholamines (Gerich *et al* 1979; Rizza *et al* 1979; Gerich 1988). Breastfed term infants do generally have lower blood glucose concentrations than those artificially fed but they do have higher blood ketone body concentrations and so are able to mount a greater ketogenic response to hypoglycaemia (Hawdon *et al* 1992). Therefore, providing the midwife is assured that the infant is full term and healthy and the weight is appropriate for gestation, there is no reason why these infants should not breastfeed on demand without giving rise to concern for their blood glucose status. In order to facilitate successful breastfeeding and to protect against clinical dehydration the midwife must be involved in the giving of breastfeeding advice soon after delivery. Appropriate teaching may include explanations regarding the composition of colostrum and mature milk, the newborn baby's requirement during the early postnatal period, the importance of hindmilk and the unrestricted duration of feeds (RCM 1991).

Transient hypoglycaemia may also occur as a result of decreased production of glucose; the following are examples of this decreased production:

Prematurity The preterm infant is particularly susceptible to hypoglycaemia for a number of reasons. The stores of glycogen in the liver are accrued in the latter part of pregnancy so the preterm infant has incomplete reserves at birth. The high neonatal glucose requirement quickly depletes the glycogen stores and renders the infant susceptible. In addition, other contributory factors which may predispose preterm infants to hypoglycaemia include the functional immaturity of digestive, glycogenolytic and glucogenic processes and the potential problems of hypothermia and asphyxia.

Birth asphyxia Infants who are stressed *in utero* or at the time of delivery are at risk of hypoglycaemia. Hypoxia and acidosis lead to increased catecholamine activity which promotes hepatic glycogenolysis, a process which depletes the stores of glycogen. Following asphyxia the neonate relies largely on anaerobic metabolism for energy production, but this process requires more glucose and, as a result, glucose from lipolysis and glycogenolysis is rapidly consumed.

Sepsis Hypoglycaemia has been reported in some infants with sepsis. A study in 1981 reported that septic infants had an increased rate of glucose utilisation (Leake *et al* 1981). This stimulation of glucose may be as a result of circulating endotoxins which increase the rate of glycolysis. In addition, increased catecholamine levels in response to the stress of acute infection play a part, as will pyrexia and an increased metabolic rate. Blood glucose monitoring, therefore, is an essential component of the management of the infant with sepsis.

Hypothermia Hypothermia may result in hypoglycaemia following delivery due to the rapid depletion of brown fat used for nonshivering thermogenesis. The infants most at risk are those who are unable to support their own glucose requirements.

Small for gestational age (SGA) The cause of hypoglycaemia in these infants appears to be multifactorial. Glycogen stores are decreased and there is also impaired gluconeogenesis. Metabolic demands are increased and these infants, whether preterm or growth-retarded, have an increased ratio of surface area to body mass, which increases the amount of energy needed for thermoregulation. In addition, infants with asymmetric growth retardation have an increased ratio of brain to body mass, which results in cerebral glucose requirements out of proportion to the liver's ability to respond. A recent study reported the frequency of hypoglycaemia in these infants to be 14.7 per cent and the mean time at which hypoglycaemia occurred was 6.1 hours of age. This particular study suggested that screening for hypoglycaemia in SGA infants should continue for 48 hours following delivery (Holtrop 1993).

☐ **Transient hypoglycaemia – increased disappearance of glucose due to transient increased circulating insulin levels**

Infant of a poorly controlled diabetic mother Prior to delivery the fetus becomes hyperglycaemic as a result of increased transfer of glucose across the placenta from the hyperglycaemic mother. The fetal pancreatic beta cells are stimulated by the increased fetal glucose concentration to produce abnormally high levels of insulin. *In utero* the increase in cellular glucose uptake is equalled by the increased insulin secretion. Following delivery, however, the source of glucose is suddenly removed while the hyperinsulinism persists resulting in hypoglycaemia. The persistent high levels of circulating insulin *in utero* have effects on all insulinsensitive tissues giving rise to the myriad of clinical signs and symptoms seen in these infants – for example, macrosomia, congenital malformations, fetal distress, sudden fetal death, hypocalcaemia, respiratory distress and feeding difficulties.

Maternal glucose infusions Fetal hyperinsulinism and neonatal hypoglycaemia may be caused by the administration of intravenous fluids containing glucose to women in the 2–3 hours prior to delivery (Kenepp *et al* 1982; Grylack *et al* 1984).

Maternal drugs The majority of drugs given to pregnant women cross the placenta and can have an effect on the fetus. Betasympathomimetics, commonly used in the prophylaxis of preterm labour (for example ritodrine), have occasionally been associated with neonatal hypoglycaemia (Epstein *et al* 1979; Procianoy & Pinheiro 1982). This may be due to both direct fetal insulin secretion as well as effects mediated via abnormal glucose concentrations. Propranolol may also induce hypoglycaemia via inhibition of catecholamine-induced glycogenolysis.

Beckwith-Wiedemann syndrome This condition is associated with pancreatic beta cell hyperplasia and hyperinsulinism. The syndrome is characterised by exomphalos, macroglossia, macrosomia and hypoglycaemia (Roberton 1992).

Erythroblastosis fetalis There is a well recognised association between hypoglycaemia and rhesus incompatibility. The hypoglycaemia is due to hyperinsulinaemia, although the pathophysiology is not fully understood (Roberton 1992).

Polycythaemia This is due to a direct result of increased glucose consumption by the red cell mass as well as secondary effects on the intestinal absorption of substrates (Roberton 1992).

☐ **Persistent or recurrent hypoglycaemia**

These are generally less common causes of neonatal hypoglycaemia and these disease states represent hormone excess or enzyme deficiency. Most of them are associated with hyperinsulinism and their control and outcome is somewhat dependent on how rapidly the diagnosis is made. They include – insulin producing tumours such as nesidioblastoma; leucine sensitivity; isolated growth hormone deficiency; cortisol deficiency; and inborn errors of metabolism or hereditary defects in metabolism such as galactosaemia or glycogen storage disease.

■ **Antenatal management and parentcraft teaching**

The midwife can have a direct influence on the careful monitoring of 'high risk' pregnancies from an early stage and she may therefore be in a position to reduce to some degree the likelihood of some of these infants developing hypoglycaemia. At the initial booking visit the midwife has the opportunity, whilst taking the maternal history, to evaluate whether the infant may be at risk. In addition to checking for any diabetes mellitus or hypoglycaemia, she should also check for the following:

● Blood group incompatibility;
● Metabolic disorders/disease;
● Previous poor obstetric history;
● Any unexplained stillbirth;
● Pre-eclampsia or hypertension;
● Any pre-existing maternal disease;
● Smoking or alcohol consumption;
● Any history of previous or current maternal drug exposure, (chlorpropamide, benzothiazides, propranolol, steroids).

Throughout the pregnancy the midwife will be monitoring the mother and her fetus for any signs which may predispose to the necessity of an early delivery. This will be particularly pertinent if there is a multiple pregnancy or if there have been any concerns regarding the growth and wellbeing of the fetus.

■ Prompt identification and recognition of infants 'at risk'

At the time of delivery the midwife must be aware that hypoglycaemia has been reported in infants whose mothers have received beta-sympathomimetic drugs such as ritodrine or salbutamol (Epstein *et al* 1979; Ogata 1981; Procianoy & Pinheiro 1982) for the prevention of preterm labour. The study of Epstein (1979) described five infants with hypoglycaemia, three of whom were symptomatic following maternal treatment with beta-agonists. The risk of hypoglycaemia appeared to be higher if the drug had been discontinued less than two days before delivery. In addition, inappropriate fluid management during labour may lead to transient hypoglycaemia (Kenepp *et al* 1982; Grylack *et al* 1984). Both these studies reported that if >25 grams per hour of dextrose was given in the two hours prior to delivery, there was a greater than fivefold increase in the risk of developing neonatal hypoglycaemia. In all instances anticipation and recognition are the most important steps in preventing hypoglycaemia. In those infants deemed to be 'at risk', the midwife has a responsibility to take all the steps she can to ensure that the infant has the optimum chance to maintain normoglycaemia. This will involve ensuring that a neutral thermal environment is maintained in order to minimise energy expenditure. Obviously if at all possible any degree of asphyxia must be avoided, however if this does occur the midwife must then initiate the necessary and appropriate observations and management. Often this particular group of infants has unusually high glucose requirements (Bhowmick & Lewandowski 1989) and it can be difficult to ensure these requirements are met as these infants may be fluid restricted in order to minimise any cerebral oedema.

Once delivery has taken place and accurate Apgar scores have been recorded, the midwife then has the opportunity to assess the infant clinically. It is important not only to record the clinical observations (weight, length, head circumference) but also to correlate these findings with the gestational age of the infant to establish whether the infant is small for gestational age. Whilst undertaking these observations, the midwife can also examine the baby in more detail. Any abnormal findings such as signs of increased adiposity or polycythaemia must be reported. Having identified those infants 'at risk', the subsequent monitoring and management of the infant and family is of paramount importance. It is, therefore, the responsibility of the midwife to ensure that adequate enteral feeding is initiated soon after birth and that caloric usage is minimised by decreasing environmental stress.

During the daily examination of the infant the midwife will be able to evaluate the infant for any of the clinical manifestations of hypoglycaemia (Lilien *et al* 1991; Roberton 1992):

- Apathy and hypotonia;
- Abnormal cry;
- Feeding difficulties;
- Tremor, 'jitteriness';
- Cyanosis;
- Tachypnoea;
- Irritability;
- Temperature instability;
- Convulsions.

It is clear that most of the above symptoms are non-specific and may have a different aetiology, however hypoglycaemia should always be suspected as there is no doubt that the implications of hypoglycaemia in relation to long term outcome are of great significance. Clinical signs are usually alleviated immediately with concomitant correction of the glucose level.

■ Screening methods and diagnosis

In most clinical settings the most common initial screening method used by midwives and nurses would be reagent strips. These test strips produce a colour change that varies depending on the amount of glucose present in the drop of blood on the strip. These methods, although used regularly, should be seen purely as an initial screening test and if an abnormal result is found then this must be checked immediately using a standard laboratory method. Several studies (Perelman *et al* 1982; Herrera & Hsiang 1983; Conrad *et al* 1989; Holtrop *et al* 1990) have reported the inaccuracy of test strips and also that they demonstrate only a modest correlation with actual blood glucose concentrations measured in laboratories. In some instances, use of the test strips in isolation would have resulted in the missed diagnosis of moderate to severe hypoglycaemia in some infants. The false negative rate with the test strips ranged from 11–17 per cent depending on the product used. In a recent study 12 infants were diagnosed as hypoglycaemic using BM stix, of these 12 infants, four were subsequently found to have blood glucose concentrations well within the normal range (Hawdon *et al* 1992). In order to achieve as accurate a result as possible the following points should be remembered.

1. The strips must be in date otherwise the readings may be lower than the actual value.
2. Capillary samples from unwarmed heels may lead to underestimation, this is due to stasis.
3. A large drop of blood must remain on the test strip for the appropriate time.
4. If any isopropyl alcohol from the swabs used remains on the heel after the test has been performed the result may be falsely elevated (Grazaitis & Sexson 1980).
5. Any infant with polycythaemia must have the plasma and not the whole blood concentration measured on the test strips as there is a decrease in the blood glucose level recorded with increased packed-cell volume (Dacombe *et al* 1981).

In conclusion, if hypoglycaemia is suspected on the basis of reagent strip measurement, it is imperative that this is checked and confirmed in a laboratory. In the interim, however, treatment for hypoglycaemia should be initiated.

■ Strategies of treatment

The management of neonatal hypoglycaemia includes the early identification of infants 'at risk', the initiation of enteral milk feeds and the minimisation of caloric usage by decreasing environmental stress.

□ Enteral feeds

If it is possible, and if the infant is asymptomatic, then the first line of treatment would be to increase the volume of enteral feeds. The carbohydrate content in breast milk is superior to that of formula milk and the calories, particularly in hindmilk, may be sufficiently high in fat to make an important contribution to the energy value of the feed (Lucas *et al* 1979). Therefore, if the mother is breastfeeding, the midwife must ensure that the mother is aware of the importance of correct positioning, that the duration of feeds is unrestricted and the importance of allowing the baby to finish spontaneously at each breast so enabling the milk which contains the most calories to be consumed (RCM 1991). If the infant is sleepy or is not able to feed either at the breast or by bottle, then alternative methods of feeding should be tried, for example cup and spoon or via a nasogastric tube (Lang *et al* 1994). If after optimising the enteral milk intake hypoglycaemia still poses a problem, then intravenous glucose must be commenced.

☐ **Intravenous therapy**

A recent study confirmed that intravenous glucose treatment administered at a constant rate of 5 mg/kg/min (= 72 mls/kg/day) 10 per cent dextrose adequately corrected hypoglycaemia without a disproportionate increase in plasma insulin concentrations (Hawdon *et al* 1994). In addition to the infusion, enteral feeds should be continued if at all possible and when appropriate there should be a gradual decrease in the amount of intravenous fluids with a concurrent increase in enteral feeds. In the past it was common for infants to receive a glucose bolus of 0.25–0.5 g/kg given as dextrose 25 per cent followed by a continuous infusion. However, such large boluses have been associated with increased pancreatic insulin secretion producing rebound hyper- or hypoglycaemia (Lilien *et al* 1980). It was also recognised that the boluses inhibit glucagon secretion (Girard 1990) and that high concentrations of glucose are hypertonic and can cause severe damage to fragile neonatal veins, perhaps resulting in extravasation.

If there is still no response then other agents must be used. Controversy remains concerning the optimum choice of first line management for some infants (Hawdon *et al* 1994; Mehta 1994), however the following may be considered suitable.

Glucagon Glucagon can be administered intravenously or intramuscularly if an intravenous line cannot be swiftly sited. This injection of glucagon will release glycogen from hepatic stores and has been found to be effective in infants of diabetic mothers but it is of less benefit in infants who have growth retardation or are SGA as they have poor glycogen stores (Carter *et al* 1988). The glucagon is usually given as an intravenous bolus followed by an intravenous infusion of 10 per cent dextrose. This is to counteract the risk of increased insulin secretion in response to the surge of glucose produced as a result of the glucagon. If these initial measures are not sufficient other forms of treatment may be necessary.

Diazoxide Diazoxide also suppresses insulin release and has been suggested as a treatment for extreme hypoglycaemia due to hyperinsulinaemia (Mehta *et al* 1987).

Somatostatin Somatostatin inhibits release of both insulin and glucagon but the natural hormone has a very short life. It is usually used as a means of short term stabilisation (Kirk *et al* 1988) for those infants who have islet cell dysplasia who will eventually require surgery, although others have suggested it may be used as definite therapy (Jackson *et al* 1987; Wilson *et al* 1988).

Steroids The use of steroids, in particular hydrocortisone, may improve the hypoglycaemia by decreasing peripheral glucose utilisation and enhancing the response to glucagon (Sann *et al* 1979). However, their use should be limited owing to the several side-effects which may be encountered by the infant who may already be in a vulnerable state.

□ **Oral lipid supplementation**

Enteral administration of medium chain triglyceride (MCT) has been shown to have a glycaemic effect in infants who were not enterally fed (Sann *et al* 1981; 1982; 1988). However, the results of a more recent study (Hawdon *et al* 1994) did not confirm these findings and the increases which occurred in blood glucose, ketone body concentrations and in glucose production rates were all less than those reported by Sann and colleagues in 1982.

■ **Long term sequelae and outcome following hypoglycaemia**

Although the definition, significance and management of hypoglycaemia remains under discussion, the long term outcome in term infants does appear to be related to the severity and duration of the hypoglycaemia. In older studies, infants of diabetic mothers had a higher incidence of neurodevelopmental abnormalities than normal neonates, but this finding has not been supported by more recent studies (Persson & Gentz 1984). There is now however, clear evidence that glucose is essential for normal brain cell function and that neonatal hypoglycaemia may result in damage to both neuronal and glial cells, the consequence of which may be severe handicap or even death. One of the earliest reports of neurological complications following hypoglycaemia was in 1959. Of eight infants who had severe symptomatic hypoglycaemia, two became spastic and mentally retarded (Cornblath *et al* 1959). Since that time several other studies have confirmed that symptomatic hypoglycaemia can cause irreversible neural damage (Haworth & Coadin 1960; Brown & Wallis 1963). However, the short and long term consequences were until recently not well established in those infants who were classified as 'asymptomatic'. There is little doubt that neonatal neurological outcome following seizures is poor (Pildes *et al* 1974), however the long term development and outcome of infants who were 'asymptomatic' has been a controversial issue (Haworth & McRae 1965; Koivisto *et al* 1972; Pildes *et al* 1974; Volpe 1986). Two of these studies (Haworth & McRae 1965; Koivisto *et al* 1972) have since been criticised. Both studies had very short follow-up periods (8–30 months) when compared with the study by Pildes *et al* (5–7 years), which suggested that it may take many years for any differences to become apparent. Other studies have investigated the effects of hypoglycaemia on neurological function using the electroencephalogram (EEG), this, however, is a non-specific measure of brain function. A more recent study (Koh *et al* 1988b) evaluated neural function using evoked potentials in children, some of whom were symptomatic and some who were asymptomatic during periods of hypoglycaemia. (Koh and colleagues defined hypoglycaemia as a blood glucose concentration < 2.6 mmol/l). The recording of evoked potentials allows objective serial measurements of neural function in specific neural pathways in relation to the blood glucose measurement. This study measured neural activity in the somatosensory and the auditory pathways in order to provide a sensitive index of the lowest blood glucose concentration compatible with normal neural function.

Abnormalities in evoked potentials have been used in other clinical situations and were found to be of prognostic value (Starr *et al* 1977; Wennenberg *et al* 1982), however no previous studies had related acute changes in sensory evoked potentials to the blood glucose concentration. In all those subjects whose blood glucose concentration was recorded as 2.6 mmol/l or greater, no abnormal changes in neural function were found. However, abnormal evoked potentials were recorded in 99 per cent of children whose blood glucose concentration fell below 2.6 mmol/l and 50 per cent of these were 'asymptomatic'.

The long term sequelae for preterm infants is complicated further by the fact that they are usually smaller and sicker before even developing hypoglycaemia. In a study of 661 preterm infants, Lucas and colleagues (1988) reported that hypoglycaemia (a blood glucose concentration of < 2.6 mmol/l) was found in 67 per cent of the infants. In 25 per cent of the infants the hypoglycaemia was found repeatedly on 3–30 days. Prolonged hypoglycaemia (i.e. a blood glucose concentration < 2.6 mmol/l for five days or more) was strongly related to reduced mental and motor development scores at 18 months (corrected age) and the incidence of cerebral palsy or developmental delay was increased. These results were analysed and presented after other risk factors for developmental delay were accounted for by multivariate analysis. This study has been criticised on a number of grounds, yet it does re-emphasise the importance of maintaining a blood glucose concentration of 2.6 mmol/l or greater in those vulnerable infants who are 'at risk'.

■ Recommendations for clinical practice in the light of currently available evidence

1. Effective antenatal care requires an appropriate level of expertise and experience. The midwife must try to ensure that she is fully aware of all the predisposing factors which may precipitate neonatal hypoglycaemia.
2. It is imperative that the midwife identifies 'at risk' pregnancies early. Recognition of these pregnancies is the most important factor in preventing hypoglycaemia. In providing effective antenatal care the midwife will be able to screen for abnormalities in the mother and fetus.
3. Mothers of fetuses at risk must be closely monitored during pregnancy and labour. The midwife has a major role to play in acquiring an accurate detailed history at the initial booking visit. She will then be in a position to exercise her autonomy by discussing with the prospective parents the services and facilities available for the family to ensure a healthy pregnancy.
4. This particular group of women may require the skills and expertise of a multidisciplinary team. The midwife will be

involved in initiating and planning a programme of antenatal care which will be supervised by an obstetrician.

5. Accurate clinical observations must be recorded from the initial booking visit. This will include not only a clinical assessment of the mother and fetus but also ultrasound scans, biochemical tests and antenatal cardiotocography.

6. At the time of delivery the midwife should ensure that a neutral thermal environment is maintained so ensuring that the caloric requirements of the infant are kept to a minimum.

7. Following delivery infants who are 'at risk' must be carefully assessed and monitored. The midwife must be aware of the definition of hypoglycaemia in her practice area.

8. The midwife must adopt a pragmatic, flexible approach to feeding to ensure that, if at all possible, there is no separation of mother and baby. This may include using other methods of feeding if the baby is unable to suckle, for example a cup and spoon may be used or if necessary a nasogastric tube. If the baby is breastfeeding and if hypoglycaemia persists, the paediatrician may request that extra milk – either breast milk or formula milk – be given.

9. Any borderline or abnormal blood results found on reagent strips must be reported to a paediatrician and further laboratory analysis undertaken.

▪ Practice check

- Is there a specific policy in your practice area for identifying 'at risk' infants antenatally?
- What definition of hypoglycaemia is used in your maternity unit?
- Is this definition used for all infants irrespective of the antenatal history, condition at birth, gestation and weight?
- Is there a protocol for the management of hypoglycaemia in your maternity unit? Is it based on sound research?
- Are 'at risk' infants specifically monitored following delivery? Does this monitoring involve regular estimations of blood glucose concentrations and a predetermined feeding protocol?
- Who is responsible for the supervision and monitoring of these infants – should it be the midwife or the paediatrician?

- Which screening methods are used to detect hypoglycaemia in your unit? How suitable are they?
- Are the midwives and doctors who use them aware of the limitations of these methods?
- Is it routine in your unit for infants who have suffered hypoglycaemia to have long term follow-up?

■ References

Bhowmick SK, Lewandowski L 1989 Prolonged hyperinsulinaemia and hypoglycaemia in an asphyxiated small for gestation infant: case management and literature review. Clinical Pediatrics (Philadelphia) 28: 575–8

Bozzetti P, Ferrarri MM, Marconi AM 1988 The relationship of maternal and fetal glucose concentrations in the human from midgestation until term. Metabolism 37: 358–63

Brown RJK, Wallis PG 1963 Hypoglycaemia in the newborn infant. Lancet i: 1278–81

Carter PE, Lloyd DJ, Duffy P 1988 Glucagon for hypoglycaemia in infants small for gestational age. Archives of Disease in Childhood 63(10): 1264–6

Cobliner S 1911 Blutzuckeruntersuchungen bei sauglingen. Zeitschrift fur Kunder heilkunde 1: 207–16

Conrad PD, Sparks JW, Osberg I, Abrams I, Hay WW Jr 1989 Clinical application of a new glucose analyzer in the neonatal intensive care unit: comparison with other methods. Journal of Pediatrics 114: 281–7

Cornblath M, Odell GB, Levin EY 1959 Symptomatic neonatal hypoglycemia associated with toxemia of pregnancy. Journal of Pediatrics 55: 545–62

Cornblath M, Reisner SH 1965 Blood glucose in the neonate, clinical significance. New England Journal of Medicine 275: 236–43

Cornblath M, Schwartz R, Aynsley-Green A, Lloyd J 1990 Hypoglycemia in infancy: the need for a rational definition. Pediatrics 85: 834–7

Dacombe CM, Dalton RG, Goldie RJ, Osborne JP 1981 Effect of packed cell volume on blood glucose concentrations. Archives of Disease in Childhood 56: 789–91

Epstein MF, Nicholls E, Stubblefield PG 1979 Neonatal hypoglycemia after beta-sympathomimetic tocolytic therapy. Journal of Pediatrics 94: 449–53

Evans SE, Crawford JS, Stevens ID 1986 Fluid therapy for induced labour under epidural analgesia: biochemical consequences for mother and infant. British Journal of Obstetrics and Gynaecology 93: 329–33

Fluge G 1975 Neurological findings at follow-up in neonatal hypoglycaemia. Acta Paediatrica Scandinavica 64: 629–34

Frazier TE, Karl IE, Hillman LS 1981 Direct measurement gluconeogenesis $(2,3,^{13}C2)$ alanine in the human newborn. American Journal of Physiology 240: E615–21

Gerich J, Davis J, Lorenzi M *et al* 1979 Hormonal mechanisms of recovery from insulin-induced hypoglycaemia in man. American Journal of Physiology 236: E380–5

Gerich JE 1988 Glucose counterregulation and its impact on diabetes mellitus. Diabetes 37: 1606–17

Girard J 1986 Gluconeogenesis in late fetal and neonatal life. Biology of the Neonate 50: 237–58

Girard J 1990 Metabolic adaptation to change of nutrition at birth. Biology of the Neonate 58 (suppl): 3–15

Grazaitis DM, Sexson NR 1980 Erroneously high Dextrostix values caused by isopropyl alcohol. Pediatrics 66: 221

Grylack LJ, Chu SS, Scanlon JW 1984 Use of intravenous fluids before cesarean section: effects on perinatal glucose, insulin and sodium homeostasis. Obstetrics and Gynecology 63: 654–8

Hawdon JM, Ward-Platt MP 1993 Metabolic adaptation in small for gestational age infants. Archives of Disease in Childhood 68(3): 262–8

Hawdon JM, Ward-Platt MP, Aynsley-Green A 1992 Patterns of metabolic adaptation for preterm and term infants in the first neonatal week. Archives of Disease in Childhood 67: 357–65

Hawdon JM, Aynsley-Green A, Ward-Platt MP 1993a Neonatal blood glucose concentrations: metabolic effects of intravenous glucagon and intragastric medium chain triglyceride. Archives of Disease in Childhood 68: 255–61

Hawdon JM, Weddell A, Aynsley-Green A, Ward-Platt MP 1993b Hormonal and metabolic response to hypoglycaemia in small for gestational age infants. Archives of Disease in Childhood 68(3): 269–73

Hawdon JM, Ward-Platt MP, Aynsley-Green A 1994 Prevention and management of neonatal hypoglycaemia. Archives of Disease in Childhood 70: F60–5

Haworth JC, Coodin FJ 1960 Idiopathic spontaneous hypoglycemia in children. Report of seven cases and review of the literature. Pediatrics 25: 748–65

Haworth JC, McRae KN 1965 Neonatal hypoglycaemia. Canadian Medical Association Journal 92: 861–5

Hay WW Jr 1991. Neonatal nutrition and metabolism: 93–104. Mosby Year Book, St Louis

Herrera AJ, Hsiang YH 1983 Comparison of various methods of blood sugar screening in newborn infants. Journal of Pediatrics 102: 769–72

Holtrop PC, Madison KA, Kieckle FL, Karcher RE, Batton DG 1990 A comparison of chromogen strip (Chemstrip bg) and serum glucose values in newborns. American Journal of Diseases in Children 144: 183–5

Holtrop PC 1993 The frequency of hypoglycemia in full-term large and small for gestational age newborns. American Journal of Perinatology 10(2): 150–4

Jackson JA, Hahn HB, Oltrof CE, O'Dorisio TM, Vinik AL 1987 Long-term treatment of refractory neonatal hypoglycaemia with long-acting somatostatin analog. Journal of Pediatrics 111: 548–51

Kalthan SC, D'Angelo LJ, Savin SM 1979 Glucose production in pregnant women at term gestation. Journal of Clinical Investigation 63: 388–9

Kenepp NB, Shelley WC, Gabbe SG 1982 Fetal and neonatal hazards of maternal hydration with 5% dextrose before caesarean section. Lancet i: 1150–52

Kirk JMW, Di Silvio L, Hindmarsh PC, Brook CGD 1988 Somatostatin analogue in short term management of hyperinsulinism. Archives of Disease in Childhood 63: 1493–4

Koh THHG, Eyre JA, Aynsley-Green A, Tarbit M 1988a Neonatal hypoglycaemia: the controversy regarding definition. Archives of Disease in Childhood 63: 1386–8

Koh THHG, Aynsley-Green A, Tarbit M, Eyre JA 1988b Neural dysfunction during hypoglycaemia. Archives of Disease in Childhood 63: 1353–8

Koivisto M, Blanco Sequrios M, Krause U 1972 Neonatal symptomatic and asymptomatic hypoglycaemia: a follow-up study of 151 children. Developmental Medical Child Neurology 14: 603–14

Lang S, Lawrence CJ, Orme RL'E 1994 Cup feeding: an alternative method of infant feeding. Archives of Disease in Childhood 71: 365–9

Leake RD, Fiser RH, Oh W 1981 Rapid glucose disappearance in infants with infection. Clinical Pediatrics 20: 397

Lilien LD, Srinivasan G, Yeh TF, Pildes RS 1991 Hypoglycemia and hyperglycemia. In Yeh TF (ed) Neonatal therapeutics 2nd edn. Mosby Year Book, St Louis

Lilien LD, Pildes R, Srinivasan G 1980 Treatment of neonatal hypoglycaemia with minibolus and intravenous glucose infusion. Journal of Pediatrics 97: 95–8

Lucas A, Adrian TE, Aynsley-Green A, Bloom SR 1980 Iatrogenic hyperinsulinism at birth. Lancet i: 144–5

Lucas A, Lucas PJ, Baum JD 1979 Patterns of milk flow in breast-fed infants. Lancet ii: 57–8

Lucas A, Morley R, Cole TJ 1988 Adverse neurodevelopmental outcome of moderate neonatal hypoglycaemia. British Medical Journal 297: 1304–8

Marsac C 1976 Development of gluconeogenic enzymes in the liver of human newborns. Biology of the Neonate 28: 317

Mehta A, Wootton R, Cheng KL, Penfold P, Halliday D, Stacey TE 1987 Effect of diazoxide or glucagon on hepatic glucose production rate during extreme neonatal hypoglycaemia. Archives of Disease in Childhood 62: 924–30

Mehta A 1994 Prevention and management of neonatal hypoglycaemia. Archives of Disease in Childhood 70: F54–F60

Mott JC 1961 The ability of young mammals to withstand total oxygen lack. British Medical Bulletin 17: 144–8

Neligan GA, Robson E, Watson J 1963 Hypoglycaemia in the newborn. A sequel of intrauterine malnutrition. Lancet i: 1282–4

Ogata ES 1981 Isoxysuprine infusion in the rat: maternal fetal and neonatal glucose homeostasis. Journal of Perinatal Medicine 9: 293–301

Padbury J, Roberman B, Oddie TH 1981 Fetal catecholamine release in response to labor and delivery. Obstetrics and Gynecology 60: 607–11

Perelman RH, Gutcher GR, Engle MJ, MacDonald MJ 1982 Comparative analysis of four methods for rapid glucose determination in neonates. American Journal of Diseases in Children 136: 1051–3

Persson B, Gentz J 1984 Follow-up of children of insulin dependent and gestational diabetic mothers. Acta Pediatrica Scandinavica 73: 349

Pildes RS, Cornblath M, Warren I 1974 A prospective controlled study of neonatal hypoglycemia. Pediatrics 54: 5–14

Procianoy RS, Pinheiro CEA 1982 Neonatal hyperinsulinemia after short-term maternal beta-sympathomimetic therapy. Journal of Pediatrics 101: 612–14

Rizza R, Cryer P, Gerich J 1979 Role of glucagon, catecholamines and growth hormone in human glucose counterregulation: effects of somatostatin and combined alpha and beta adrenergic blockade and plasma glucose recovery and glucose flux rates following insulin-induced hypoglycaemia. Journal of Clinical Investigation 64: 62–71

Roberton NRC 1992 Textbook of neonatology 2nd edn. Churchill Livingstone, Edinburgh

Royal College of Midwives 1991 Successful breastfeeding 2nd edn. RCM, London

Sann L, Ruiton A, Mathieu M, Lashe Y 1979 Effects of intravenous hydrocortisone administration on glucose homeostasis in small-for-gestational age infants. Acta Paediatrica Scandinavica 68: 113–18

Sann L, Mathieu M, Lasne Y, Ruitton A 1981 Effect of oral administration of lipids with 67% medium chain triglycerides on glucose homeostasis in pattern neonates. Metabolism 30: 712–16

Sann L, Divy P, Lasne Y, Ruitton A 1982 Effect of oral lipid administration on glucose homeostasis in small for gestational age infants. Acta Paediatrica Scandinavica 71: 923–7

Sann L, Mousson B, Rousson M, Maire I, Bethenod M 1988 Prevention of neonatal hypoglycaemia by oral lipid supplementation in low birth weight infants. European Journal of Pediatrics 147(2): 158–61

Sedgwick JP, Ziegler MR 1920 The nitrogenous and sugar content of the blood of the newborn. American Journal of Disease in Children 19: 429–32

Spence JC 1921 Some observations on sugar tolerance with special reference to variations found at different ages. Quarterly Journal of Medicine 14: 314–26

Srinivasan G, Pildes R, Cattamanchi G, Voora S, Lilien LD 1986 Plasma glucose levels in normal neonates: a new look. Journal of Pediatrics 109: 114–17

Starr A, Amlie RN, Martin WH, Sansers S 1977 Development of auditory function in newborn infants revealed by auditory brain stem potentials. Pediatrics 60: 831–9

Volpe JJ 1986 Neurology of the newborn. WB Saunders, Philadelphia

Wennberg, RP, Ahlfors CE, Bickers R, McMurty CA, Shelter JL 1982 Abnormal auditory brainstem response in a newborn infant with hyperbilirubinemia: improvement with exchange transfusion. Journal of Pediatrics 100: 624–6

Widstrom AM, Ranso-Arvidson AB, Christensson K, Mattieson AS, Winberg J, Vvnas-Moberg K 1987 Gastric suction in healthy newborn infants. Acta Paediatrica Scandinavica 76: 566–72

Wilson DC, Carson DJ, Quinn RJ 1988 Long-term use of somatostatin analogue SMS 201–995 in the treatment of hypoglycaemia due to nesidioblastosis. Acta Paediatrica Scandinavica 77: 467–70

Zimmer EZ, Goldstein I, Feldman E 1986 Maternal and newborn levels of glucose, sodium and osmolality after preloading with three intravenous solutions during elective caesarean sections. European Journal of Obstetrics, Gynaecology and Reproductive Biology 23: 61–5

■ Suggested further reading

Polk DH 1991 Disorders of carbohydrate metabolism. In Taeusch HW, Ballard RA, Avery MG (eds) Schaffer and Avery's Diseases of the Newborn 6th edn: 965–71. WB Saunders, Philadelphia

Cornblath M, Schwartz R 1991 Hypoglycemia in the neonate. In Cornblath M, Schwartz R (eds) Disorders of carbohydrate metabolism in infancy. WB Saunders, Philadelphia

Aynsley-Green A, Soltez G 1992 Disorders of blood glucose homeostasis in the neonate. In Roberton NRC (ed) Neonatology: 777–98. Churchill Livingstone, Edinburgh

Lilien LD, Srinivasan G, Yeh TF, Pildes RS 1991 Hypoglycemia and hyperglycemia. In Yeh TF (ed) Neonatal therapeutics 2nd edn. Mosby Year Book, St Louis

Aynsley-Green A, Soltesz G 1992 Metabolic and endocrine disorders. In Roberton NRC (ed) Textbook of neonatology: 777–97 Churchill Livingstone, Edinburgh

Chapter 9

Routine clinical care in the immediate postnatal period

Sally Marchant and Jo Garcia

This chapter aims to look at the clinical components of the care given by midwives to postnatal women. The postnatal daily examination requires the midwife to observe and record the state of health and recovery of the postnatal mother. The form this examination takes has become a routine midwifery procedure described in standard textbooks. There has been little, if any, evaluation of the value that this form of care has for the majority of women.

The chapter reports some results of a study which looked in depth at the postnatal care of nearly 200 women. Data describing the composition of the postnatal checks for these women in the first 12 days after the birth of the baby are used to explore whether routines are applied in practice.

The potential effectiveness of the individual components of routine clinical care is then examined by looking at one aspect of the postnatal check – assessment of uterine involution. The chapter ends with suggestions for future research.

■ **It is assumed that you are already aware of the following:**

- The physiology of the puerperium;
- The most common problems resulting in morbidity for the postnatal mother;
- The statutory responsibility of the midwife in the postnatal period.

■ Routine examination of the postnatal mother

In this section we will look at the limited research information that we have about current practice, and at the description of this aspect of midwifery care in three current textbooks.

A Scottish study by Murphy-Black (1989) about postnatal care at home identified the physical, educational and psychosocial content of the community midwife's visit. Some tasks were reported by over 80 per cent of the mothers in Murphy-Black's study; these included checking the abdomen, examining the baby, discussing feeding, checking the mother's temperature, letting the mother talk about herself and taking the baby's temperature. Less than 20 per cent reported that the midwife took their blood pressure, helped with feeding the baby, or showed how to change a nappy, make up a bottle feed or bath the baby. Murphy-Black found that there were few systematic differences in the tasks carried out for different categories of mother. The care received by first time mothers, and those with an instrumental or operative delivery, did not differ from the average. Women who bottle fed, however, did differ from those who were breast-feeding at all in some interesting ways; for bottle feeding mothers, midwives were reported to be less likely to examine the baby or to let the mother talk, in addition to some more expected differences in practices such as checking the breasts.

Murphy-Black concluded that the midwives taking part in that study generally did not adjust their care to take account of the type of delivery or the mother's previous experiences of childbirth but tended instead to follow a routine related to the number of postnatal days on discharge from hospital. The baseline for care appeared to be focused on the midwives' rather than the mothers' perception of need.

In another Scottish study, Marsh and Sargent (1991) looked at factors which affected the duration of each visit from the community midwife and described the components of 783 postnatal visits to 224 mothers by 24 midwives. The detailed aspects of the physical check of mother and baby were not covered in this study, so there cannot be a direct comparison with the results of Murphy-Black. The authors did investigate whether aspects of the mother's health and circumstances (as recorded by the midwife) were related to the duration of each visit. Problems with feeding were associated with visits that were a fifth longer on average, and complications at delivery were associated with visits that were 12 per cent longer. Other maternal health and social problems, such as absence of family support, were not associated with the length of the visit.

Midwifery textbooks have traditionally combined a scientific approach, obstetrically based, with midwifery skills and knowledge (Leap 1993). Information on postnatal care in most standard textbooks is a good example of this combination of art and science. A knowledge of anatomy and physiology in the puerperium is needed in order for the midwife to interpret the clinical observations and to distinguish between normal and pathological conditions. An awareness of the social and psychological effects the birth might have for the family is also relevant.

We looked at three textbooks commonly used in midwifery education: *Myles Textbook for Midwives* (12th edition 1993, ed. Bennett and Brown), *Mayes' Midwifery* (11th edition 1988, ed. Sweet) and *The Art and Science of Midwifery* (1993, Silverton). Each has chapters on postnatal care which address the physical, psychological and social aspects of the care for mother and family. Two of the textbooks were recently considerably revised from a traditional format started in the 1950s; the third is a new book. All three follow a similar format which looks at the role of the midwife in postnatal care as well as giving specific clinical information and teaching on the skills required to assess the health of the postnatal mother. Comparing the actual components of the postnatal check in each of the books, all three have the same contents for the examination and, although they vary slightly in format, the components of the check are identified in all three in the form of a list. Silverton has a more discursive style and she includes more in the way of general advice for the postnatal period; the other two books deal with this material under separate headings.

An example of the suggested format for the physical examination is taken from the chapter by Ball (1993) on 'Physiology, psychology and management of the puerperium' (Bennett and Brown; pp. 241–2). 'Each day the midwife should carry out an examination of the mother, observing her general health and noting her physical and emotional well-being.' There follows a list of the main aspects of the examination, such as temperature, lochia, legs and so on, with a short description of what would be considered normal, and the possible abnormalities and appropriate action.

The current midwifery training curriculum is outlined in the *Midwives' Rules* (UKCC 1993). Apart from covering anatomy and physiology of the postnatal period, the midwife is encouraged to look at changes and developments in the puerperium as part of a complete picture rather than isolated events. The textbooks suggest that the midwife carries out a formal review of the mother and baby on a frequent basis, initially daily, or regularly throughout the first ten days and then infrequently if required at all until the twenty eighth day when care is transferred to the health visitor.

How is the material from textbooks and the *Midwives' Rules* used in training? We do not know how information is passed on, for example in a formal educational setting to student midwives. Midwifery textbooks are primarily designed to meet the needs of student midwives, but we know little about what is actually taught outside of the curriculum requirements.

Teaching, on a formal or informal basis, can take place in different locations such as the midwifery education department, the maternity hospital and the community. Qualified midwives undertake a mentor role for student midwives in a clinical setting where teaching may be more from clinical experience than theory. An ethnographic study of the experiences of student midwives identified that in the early phases of midwifery training, undertaking routine observations assumed importance probably because this represents something familiar to those from a nursing background (Davies 1990). This study also identifies some rigidity in the behaviour and attitudes of those midwives who came into contact with the students. There is the potential for conflicting information where students may be informed academically of one style of care but observe different practices in the clinical setting. This may mean questioning routine practices in some circumstances or being unclear why routine practices were not being followed in another.

Using the postnatal check format, midwives are seeking to exclude problems and yet despite significant morbidity there has been very little research into the health of postnatal women overall. Research into problems in the postnatal period has tended to be fragmented and focused on specific issues rather than how these relate. There has been a great deal of research about breastfeeding and associated problems (for example, Inch & Renfrew 1989) but little about breast inflammation, commonly known as mastitis. There has also been research into perineal pain (Sleep 1991; see also the chapter in this volume by Jennifer Sleep) and postnatal depression (for example, Romito 1989; Levy 1994). The early days of the postnatal period and the role of the midwife at this time has received little attention, however. This means that routine observations such as those of the lochia and fundal height have never been evaluated in terms of effectiveness in preventing maternal morbidity.

In addition there is a need to assess whether care should be applied as a routine to all women or whether it should be adjusted to the needs of individuals. Applying the same postnatal examination to all women, regardless of circumstances, may be wasteful of resources and less useful to women than an individualised approach. On the other hand there may be advantages in a routine approach, for example, for women who are less likely to seek help when they need it.

One aim of our study, described below, was to look at how care is being applied in practice.

■ The Postnatal Care (PNC) Project

The National Perinatal Epidemiology Unit (NPEU) Postnatal Care Project was a descriptive study designed to look at the care given to postnatal women for the first eight weeks following the birth. It investigated the care and support women expected to receive after the birth from professionals, from family and friends and then at what care they actually received. Information was collected from 192 mothers in two English health districts using semi-structured interviews, a one page calendar to record information about basic aspects of health and about home visits from midwives for the first two weeks, four diaries and a final postal questionnaire. Mothers were asked to fill in diaries every four days until the twelfth day to record the events of the early postnatal days in more detail. When the baby was about eight weeks old, women were asked to look back on their experiences. In this way we have some record of the work of the midwives who cared for these mothers during this time and some insight into whether the needs identified by mothers were being met. Midwives were also asked for their views on specific elements of the postnatal check, relating it to their usual practice.

■ Results of the PNC Project

□ Details of care expected and reported by mothers

Women recruited to the study were interviewed in hospital within 48 hours of delivery. At this time we asked women about their expectations of the midwifery care they would receive both in hospital and once they were home. Once the women had been recruited to the study and the first interview was completed, they were asked to fill in a diary at intervals of four days; on the first or second postnatal day, on day four, day eight and finally on day twelve. In this way we hoped to have a more detailed account of the physical health of the mother and baby, and any social and emotional problems. The diaries were also a way of recording midwifery care in hospital and at home.

In answers to questions about expectations of care in the first interview, almost all the mothers said that a midwife would examine them while they were in hospital (177/187, 95 per cent). Those women who thought that they would be examined were then asked:

> What do you think the midwife will include when she examines you?

Table 9.1 shows the responses which were entered by the interviewer onto a prepared list, unseen by the respondent, along with any comments made by the mother at the time.

Women in both districts had broadly similar expectations of what a midwife would be checking or asking about in the first few days after the birth. It is surprising that only about a quarter of the women included an assessment of their vaginal loss, whereas two thirds expected the midwife to record their blood pressure. In the first 48 hours after delivery, the mother may still be patterned to observations which were important in pregnancy, and regular checks will have been made of the blood pressure, although this might be less important in the puerperium. Twice as many

Table 9.1 Mothers' expectations of the content of the midwives' examination at first interview (less than 48 hours post delivery)

	District One		District Two	
	N	(%)	*N*	(%)
Temperature	59	(62)	42	(42)
Pulse	22	(23)	14	(16)
Blood pressure	65	(68)	52	(61)
Breasts	40	(42)	18	(21)
Uterus	61	(64)	42	(49)
Stitches	61	(64)	44	(52)
Vaginal loss	22	(23)	25	(29)
C/S scar	13	(14)	6	(7)
How they are feeling	45	(47)	36	(42)
Appetite	2	(2)	2	(2)
Sleep	5	(5)	0	(0)
Total	N = 95		N = 85	

Table 9.2 Mothers' recording of the content of the midwife's postnatal examination while they were in hospital

	District One		District Two	
	N	(%)	N	(%)
Temperature	142	(98)	58	(94)
Pulse	139	(96)	53	(85)
Blood pressure	118	(81)	56	(90)
Breasts	89	(61)	32	(52)
Nipples	83	(57)	28	(47)
Womb	102	(70)	33	(53)
Legs	97	(67)	38	(61)
Blood loss	123	(85)	36	(58)
Passing urine without problem	132	(91)	42	(68)
Bowels working normally	110	(76)	32	(52)
Total examinations reported	145		62	

mothers in District One (42 per cent) said that they expected some examination of their breasts compared to the mothers in District Two (21 per cent).

Turning now to the clinical care recorded by the mothers in the diaries, the mothers in hospital almost all reported being examined by a midwife that day (between 87 per cent and 94 per cent depending on the day). Table 9.2 shows the items in the midwifery examination in hospital reported by the mothers in the diary, on a checklist.

In the diaries women also recorded details of the examinations by a midwife at home. If a midwife visited at home, she usually examined the mother. On 16 occasions out of 210 (8 per cent) this did not happen. The small number of visits by a midwife at 12 days after the birth were less likely to include an examination of the mother. If a woman did have an examination she was asked to fill in what the midwife had checked using a list in the diary. Table 9.3 illustrates this.

The data in Tables 9.2 and 9.3 give us some idea about the compliance of the midwives with the standard teaching about the postnatal daily check. We will look first at care in hospital. Over 75 per cent of women in District One reported that midwives had checked six out of the ten items listed in this question in the diary. For District Two this was true of only three out of the ten items. Midwives in District Two appear to be checking routinely for a more limited list of items. The further analysis of the study data that is taking place will indicate whether the other parts of the check are being used selectively for particular women.

Table 9.3 Mothers' recording of the content of the midwife's examination when they were at home

| | District One | | District Two | |
	N	**(%)**	**N**	**(%)**
Temperature	17	(15)	60	(71)
Pulse	27	(24)	52	(61)
Blood pressure	21	(19)	45	(53)
Breasts	70	(62)	64	(75)
Nipples	57	(50)	47	(55)
Womb	79	(70)	61	(72)
Legs	71	(63)	5	(6)
Blood loss	97	(86)	65	(76)
Passing urine without problem	96	(85)	71	(84)
Bowels working normally	98	(87)	71	(84)
	N = 113		N = 85	

In both districts the midwives appeared to check the breasts and nipples less often than other items on the standard list. This is most likely to reflect that midwives do not check the breasts or nipples of women who are not breastfeeding.

In the community, midwives seem more likely to omit some items of the check altogether. The mothers' records of the midwives' observations show a greater variation between the two districts. There is a marked difference between observations of temperature, pulse and blood pressure with midwives in District Two carrying out more than twice as many observations as midwives in District One. Again in our analysis we will explore the extent to which parts of the examination are applied to particular mothers.

Going back to the first interview, women were asked a rather broader question about what they expected the midwife to do during home visits. Table 9.4 lists the frequency of tasks identified by respondents. Again an open question, rather than a list, was used. In other words they were not asked about the specific parts of a postnatal check and the categories were unseen by the respondents but marked in by the interviewer.

It is interesting that women in both Districts had similar expectations despite coming from different cultural and social environments. The majority of mothers expected the midwife to be checking their health and their baby's health on a regular basis but fewer had expectations of other things that the midwife might do. Whereas helping with feeding was expected by approximately half of the mothers, considerably fewer mothers

Table 9.4 Mothers' answers to the question 'What do you expect her to do during the (home) visit?' Data from first interview (less than 48 hours post delivery in hospital)

| | District One | | District Two | |
	N	(%)	N	(%)
General advice: baby	25	(25)	17	(20)
mother	19	(19)	19	(23)
Weigh baby	28	(28)	16	(19)
Help with feeding	50	(50)	34	(40)
Help with problems	27	(27)	16	(19)
Check cord	13	(13)	6	(7)
Blood tests for baby	8	(8)	7	(8)
Checking baby's health	93	(93)	75	(89)
Checking mother's health	96	(96)	75	(89)
Other..	35	(35)	29	(35)
Total	N = 99		N = 84	

expected the midwife to weigh their baby and even fewer to help with care of the cord. This question was asked within 48 hours of the birth and perhaps illustrates the gap between information which health professionals provide for parents in the antenatal period in the form of parentcraft and advice leaflets and booklets, and that information being retained for the postnatal period.

In the diaries a question was asked about other aspects of postnatal wellbeing. These items are shown in Table 9.5 according to the district and whether the mothers were at home or in hospital. This identifies a range of activities carried out by midwives during their checks. The only real difference in these activities and their relation to where care took place is in the large difference recorded by the mothers of observation of feeding. In District One mothers were five times more likely to have been observed feeding in hospital than at home, and three times more likely in District Two. Fairly small differences in figures for the baby examination between hospital and home might be accounted for when a baby was checked in the mother's absence and she was unaware that this had taken place.

Part of the purpose of the survey was to describe the activities of the midwives and how the mothers viewed these activities. Although our study might suggest some reasons for why there are differences in various findings, they remain descriptions of care and no form of evaluation or effectiveness can be presumed from a study of this design. Overall these figures suggest that the standard postnatal examination is more likely to be applied

Table 9.5 Question asked about aspects of postnatal wellbeing

| | District One | | District Two | |
	Hospital (%)	Home (%)	Hospital (%)	Home (%)
Today, did the midwife:				
talk to you about feeding	61	60	58	48
examine your baby	64	87	68	91
watch you breast or				
bottle feed your baby	53	8	37	13
ask how you were feeling	84	86	87	77
ask about your appetite	15	19	21	17
ask how you were sleeping	41	49	47	42
anything else	9	11	5	6
N =	148	123	62	88

in hospital than at home. Further analysis of our data will throw some light on the decisions behind the selection of mothers for a routine check.

□ The purpose and effectiveness of the postnatal examination – the case of involution

The general postnatal examination is made up of a set of screening and diagnostic tests intended to detect problems or potential problems in the mother. Some aspects of the examination are fairly straightforward and lead to immediate advice or treatment. For example, if the perineum is painful the midwife may recommend analgesia. Other parts of the examination can lead to a series of further investigations in order to decide if treatment is required. If, for example, a mother complained of calf pain or tenderness, the midwife would normally refer her for medical opinion to exclude deep venous thrombosis.

In order to decide whether the components of the postnatal examination are likely to be effective in reducing morbidity we need to look first at what it is supposed to measure, and at what action (diagnostic or therapeutic) is likely to follow. We then need to ask if the test is measuring what it is supposed to measure, and whether there is evidence that intervention reduces the risk of the expected adverse health outcome. This is best illustrated by an example. Two elements of the routine check – measurement of the symphysis-fundus distance, and questions about the lochia – are aimed at establishing that normal progress is being made and, if not, providing early warning of uterine problems such as infection and haemorrhage. Measuring the height and feel of the uterus for signs of involution and observing the amount, colour, consistency and odour of lochia are intended to identify the presence of retained placental products and/or uterine infection.

But, the links in the chain need to be examined:

1. Does palpation (or the formal measurement of the symphysis-fundus distance) give an indication of whether involution is progressing normally?
2. Is 'poor' involution assessed by palpation associated with the presence of retained products?
3. Is 'poor' involution (however assessed) associated with subsequent morbidity?
4. Are 'abnormalities' of the lochia, detected in the early postnatal period, associated with subsequent morbidity?

What answers do we have to these questions?

1. Does palpation (or the formal measurement of the symphysis-fundus distance) give an indication of whether involution is progressing normally?
If we assume that ultrasound measurement provides an accurate assessment of uterine size, we could compare clinical measurement with ultrasound measures of uterine size postpartum. We have not found any studies which have done this. In a review of the literature on assessment of uterine involution by Montgomery and Alexander (1994), the authors consider research involving the use of ultrasonography to investigate involution in the puerperium; they found no studies which looked at the observation of involution by midwives. In the five studies reviewed there is a wide variation in the range of subjects included and the outcomes measured. It is interesting that evidence from the studies did not show that parity or baby feeding method affected the rate of uterine involution. There was, however, some evidence of a positive correlation between birthweight and uterine size. The authors suggest that further research is needed to investigate the value of anthropometric assessment of fundal height as a method of monitoring uterine involution.

2. Is 'poor' involution assessed by palpation associated with the presence of retained products?
We have not found any studies that address this question.

3. Is 'poor' involution (however assessed) associated with subsequent morbidity?

One research study investigates external measurement of the symphysis-fundus height (Bergstrom & Libombo 1992). In the study a group of 51 women with 'clinically evident' endometritis-myometritis were identified. These women were diagnosed on the basis of a fever of 38°C or more and a painful uterus. They were compared to 51 healthy women matched for age, parity and days post delivery. The symphysis-fundus distance was compared between the two groups and this showed no significant difference. The authors conclude that endometritis-myometritis does not produce significantly increased fundal height and they question the validity of the widely held opinion that there is a difference in uterine size between healthy women and those with uterine infection. Many criticisms could be made of this study. There is, for example, no information about how many observers were involved or how the symphysis-fundus distance was measured. However it remains the only study which has looked at the process of external measurement of the uterus as it relates to the detection of endometritis-myometritis and suggests no value in this practice.

4. Are 'abnormalities' of the lochia, detected in the early postnatal period, associated with subsequent morbidity?

We have not found any evidence about this.

What this series of questions shows is that there is not, at present, research evidence to support or reject the current routine midwifery practice concerned with uterine 'recovery'. The subsequent care of women with uterine problems is also fraught with uncertainty. For example, there is evidence that bleeding problems and retained products of conception do not necessarily occur together. In an early study by Malvern and colleagues (1973), 8.5 per cent of women who had dilatation and curettage for clinically significant bleeding were not found to have the histology to confirm the presence of retained products. Hertzberg and Bowie (1991) found that the presence of endometrial fluid was identified in the uterine cavity also without necessarily being associated with complications. These findings are important in relation to the diagnosis of retained placental tissue using ultrasound as they indicate possible causes of misinterpretation and false positive results.

A later study which looked at the alterations in peripheral vascular resistance of uterine arteries in the puerperium (Tekay & Jouppila 1993), gives information about the use of ultrasound in identifying normal and abnormal processes of involution. This longitudinal study describes repeated ultrasonic observations on 42 healthy postpartum women without abnormal symptoms of bleeding; 266 evaluations were collected in total. One of the findings was the presence of debris in the uterine cavity in 21 per cent of women in the first week postpartum. None of these women subsequently experienced any complications.

These studies have looked in detail at the use of ultrasound in differentiating those women who may have significant pathology from those who do not. Hertzberg and Bowie (1991), in particular, note that the appearance of retained placental debris is more varied than previously thought and although they recommend undertaking ultrasound examination before curettage, they suggest that these tests require expert interpretation.

■ Future research directions

This review of one area of the postnatal check gives some idea of the complex issues that are involved. In order to make care more soundly based, there is a need for descriptive and evaluative research. For example, there is a need to audit the current practice of midwives. Are routine checks being made on all women or are some selected? If so, which women are checked? How are postnatal assessments made and recorded? What action is taken in the event of an 'abnormal' finding?

Another approach is to look at the way that the postnatal check is actually carried out by observing the care as it takes place. How do midwives explain what they are doing? Do mothers ask questions and raise concerns? How do midwives respond to the questions mothers ask? This may help us to explore the wider value of routine care in allowing women to talk to midwives without having to make a special approach.

Other research approaches could also be employed. For example, if the purpose of checking the uterus and lochia is to detect or prevent some postnatal complications, then how many of these complications are happening? How many women are having uterine infection or secondary postpartum haemorrhage? How are they treated, by whom, and where? Did they have 'abnormal' results on any of the postnatal checks? When we know this we may be in a position to decide if either the checks or the treatments are effective.

■ Recommendations for clinical practice in the light of currently available evidence

In this chapter we have not described findings that could directly lead to clear changes in current clinical practice. There is very little research about any of the aspects of routine clinical care in the puerperium. More evidence of the extent of maternal morbidity is becoming available. In order to improve care, carrying out research and audit is crucial.

■ Practice check

• What do you know about the long term postnatal health of women in your care?
• How do you carry out the postnatal check? How consistent is your practice? Have you discussed postnatal care with your midwife colleagues?
• In carrying out a 'routine' check do you give postnatal mothers enough opportunity to talk about their own health and any other concerns they have?
• Do you know what student midwives are taught about clinical aspects of postnatal care? How does your practice compare with what student midwives are taught away from the clinical area?
• Is the current recording of postnatal observations done in a way which accurately reflects the condition of the mother and baby and is useful for future reference?
• Could you carry out a clinical audit of the various components of the postnatal check? What do you think is a priority for research in this area?

■ References

Ball J 1993 Physiology, psychology and management of the puerperium. In Bennett VR, Brown LK (eds) Myles textbook for midwives 12th edn: 234–50. Churchill Livingstone, Edinburgh

Bennett VR, Brown LK (eds) 1993 Myles textbook for midwives 12th edn. Churchill Livingstone, Edinburgh

Bergstrom S, Libombo A 1992 Puerperal measurement of the symphysis-fundus measurement distance. Gynecological and Obstetric Investigation 34: 76–8

Davies R 1990 Perspectives on midwifery: students' beginnings. In

Research and the Midwife Conference Proceedings: 37–48. University of Manchester

Hertzberg B, Bowie J 1991 Ultrasound of the postpartum uterus. Journal of Ultrasound Medicine 10: 451–6

Inch S, Renfrew M 1989 Common breastfeeding problems. In Chalmers I, Enkin M, Keirse MJNC (eds) Effective care in pregnancy and childbirth: 2, 81, 1375–89. Oxford University Press, Oxford

Leap N 1993 Textbooks of midwifery. Midwives Chronicle 106 (1266): 242–5

Levy V 1994 The maternity blues in postpartum women and postoperative patients. In Robinson S, Thomson A (eds) Midwives, research and childbirth vol 3: 147–74. Chapman & Hall, London

Malvern J, Campbell S, May P 1973 Ultrasonic scanning of the puerperal uterus following secondary postpartum haemorrhage. Journal of Obstetrics and Gynaecology of the British Commonwealth 80: 320–24

Marsh J, Sargent E 1991 Factors affecting the duration of postnatal visits. Midwifery 7(4): 177–82

Montgomery E, Alexander J 1994 Assessing postnatal uterine involution: a review and a challenge. Midwifery 10(2): 73–6

Murphy-Black T 1989. Postnatal care at home: a descriptive study of mothers' needs and the maternity services. A report for the Scottish Home and Health Department. Nursing Research Unit, University of Edinburgh

Romito P 1989 Unhappiness after childbirth. In Chalmers I, Enkin M, Keirse MJNC (eds) Effective care in pregnancy and childbirth: 2, 86, 1433–48. Oxford University Press, Oxford

Silverton L 1993 The art and science of midwifery: 433–62. Prentice Hall, London

Sleep J 1991 Perineal care: a series of five randomised controlled trials. In Robinson S, Thomson A (eds) Midwives, research and childbirth vol 2: 199–251. Chapman & Hall, London

Sweet B (ed) 1988 Mayes' midwifery: a textbook for midwives (11th edn): 240–54; 387–94. Baillière Tindall, London

Tekay A, Jouppila P 1993 A longitudinal Doppler ultrasonographic assessment of the alterations in peripheral vascular resistance of the uterine arteries and ultrasonographic findings of the involuting uterus during the puerperium. American Journal of Obstetrics and Gynecology 168: 190–98

Twaddle S, Liao X, Fyvie H 1993 An evaluation of postnatal care individualised to the needs of the woman. Midwifery 9: 154–60

United Kingdom Central Council for Nursing, Midwifery and Health Visiting 1993 Midwives' Rules. UKCC, London

Index